WHEN YOUR
HORMONES
GO HAYWIRE

D0973308

OTHER BOOKS BY PAMELA SMITH, R.D.

This book contains advice and information relating to health and medicine. It is designed for your personal knowledge and to help you be a more informed consumer of medical and health services. It is not intended to be exhaustive or to replace medical advice from your physician and should be used to supplement rather than replace regular care by your physician. Readers are encouraged to consult their physicians with specific questions and concerns.

All efforts have been made to ensure the accuracy of the information contained within this book as of the date published. The author and the publisher expressly disclaim responsibility for any adverse effects resulting from the application of the information contained herein.

WHEN YOUR HORMONES GO HAYWIRE

An Updated and Revised Edition of *Take Charge of the Change*

Solutions for Women Over 40

PAMELA SMITH, R.D.

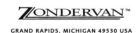

ZONDERVAN™

GRAND RAPIDS, MICHIGAN 49530 USA

ZONDERVAN™

When Your Hormones Go Haywire
Copyright © 2003, 2005 by Pamela M. Smith

Requests for information should be addressed to:
Zondervan, *Grand Rapids, Michigan 49530*

Library of Congress Cataloging-in-Publication Data

Smith, Pamela.
    [Take charge of the change]
    When your hormones go haywire : solutions for women over forty /
Pamela M. Smith.
    p. cm.
    Previously published under the title: Take charge of the change.
    Includes bibliographical references and index.
    ISBN-10: 0-310-25736-0 (softcover)
    ISBN-13: 978-0-310-25736-3
    1. Menopause—Popular works. I. Title.
RG186.S676 2005
618.1'75—dc22
                                                 2004026274
                                                            CIP

All Scripture quotations, unless otherwise indicated, are taken from the *Holy Bible: New International Version*®. NIV®. Copyright © 1973, 1978, 1984 by International Bible Society. Used by permission of Zondervan. All rights reserved.

The website addresses recommended throughout this book are offered as a resource to you. These websites are not intended in any way to be or imply an endorsement on the part of Zondervan, nor do we vouch for their content for the life of this book.

All rights reserved. No part of this publication may be reproduced, stored in a retrieval system, or transmitted in any form or by any means—electronic, mechanical, photocopy, recording, or any other—except for brief quotations in printed reviews, without the prior permission of the publisher.

Published in association with the literary agency of Ann Spangler and Company, 1420 Pontiac Road S.E., Grand Rapids, MI 49506.

Interior design by Beth Shagene

Printed in the United States of America

05 06 07 08 09 10 11 /❖DCI/ 10 9 8 7 6 5 4 3 2 1

For

Kent and Lynn Shoemaker

Your courage, your grace, your faith, and your love have
lifted me higher than can ever be measured in earthly terms.

May we ever laugh at today's troubles,
trade tomorrow's sorrows for dancing,
and celebrate this moment called now.

Contents

Thank You Notes

Forever love to Pat Martin, Jenny Phillips, Caron Loveless, Lynn Shoemaker, Arlene Deverman, Rebecca Sweatt, Mary Matthews, and Carolyn Coats—my ever-special lady-boomer friends, who have chosen to do life with me and to share all that it offers. We've laughed till we've cried and, sometimes, have just cried. I always emerge stronger and better prepared for the delights and fights each day brings.

Thank you, thank you, thank you to Ann Spangler and Linda Peterson-Kenney, who helped to bring the thought for this book into a living reality; who stole precious time from their own projects to lend input, enthusiasm, and never wavering support to mine. Ann, it was long past time to join hands and hearts; you made it happen!

Grateful thanks to Cindy Lambert, my gifted editor and new best friend, for believing and investing your pen, your heart, and immeasurable hours (hours that you did not have!) to those beliefs. To Sue Brower, for taking charge of a difficult search and coming forth with the perfect name for these words. To Verlyn Verbrugge for careful editing on a very new subject. To Cindy Davis for gifted vision in artistic direction. And to Scott Bolinder and the entire staff at Zondervan for giving me a place to share this message—and a vehicle in which to bring it forth.

Humble thanks to my clients—both person-to-person and those regular visitors to *pamsmith.com* for bringing insight, humor, honesty, and spice to this book.

Many thanks to Kent and Lynn Shoemaker and Arlene and Gary Deverman for their many instances of over-the-top generosity in providing a place of peace and creativity during the writing of this book.

Loving thanks to my husband and friend, Larry, for cheering louder and longer than everyone combined.

And thank you, Mom, Danielle, and Nicole, the ladies on either side of me, who make me the grateful one-in-the-middle. Thank you for only *silently* sighing when you ask what I am doing today, knowing that my answer is always the same. I look around and my eyes land on you, and I know that I am so very blessed. I want *you* to know—above all else—that you are incredible, you are loved immeasurably, you are my joy and my life.

INTRODUCTION

If you're like many women, you have a never-ending to-do list, a demanding job (in and/or out of the home), and a family who needs you. You often feel tired or depressed, anxious or irritable. Heart palpitations might occur often enough that you have 9-1-1 on direct dial. Or perhaps you can't sleep (although you have no problem eating!). Romance is a distant memory. Weight issues and body image struggles seem to be a way of life. Energy, peace, and purpose are sought-after treasures.

For the last twenty-five years, I have served as a nutrition and energy coach to women struggling with exactly these issues, women just like me. I've designed life strategies for young ladies who are navigating the tumultuous tween and teen years to those who are crossing the sometimes troubled waters of midlife — and for those who are seeking to add *life to their years*, not just years to their life.

My *Living Well Plan* for women has not wavered through these past two decades; it is based on strategic eating, movement, air and water, rest, as well as fostering emotional and spiritual well-being. It has expanded somewhat — to incorporate the most current research that further helps to connect the dots of how a healthy lifestyle promotes wellness in all areas of living: physically, emotionally, relationally, and spiritually. But the basics are just that — basic life principles that are not subject to a great deal of change, just enhancement as we learn more.

My goal remains helping women feel great, look great, and live great — through embracing healthy lifestyle choices and self-care. Connecting with ourselves, others, and God and properly nourishing oneself — body and soul — is critical to living well, free, and whole. Thinness is not the destination; being healthy, fit, and balanced is. The eat-right prescription is as up-to-date today as it was when I first wrote nutrition guidelines for my patient practice, later released as *Eat Well, Live Well* in the early 1990s.

So what *has* changed?

First, I have. When I started this guide to hormone balance, I was forty-seven and in the foyer of menopause. Now, as I update and add to it, I am forty-nine and sitting squarely in menopause's living room. As you read this, you may be in the same place, or perhaps just peeking in the window or on its front porch. We are not alone.

There are more than twenty million baby boomers just like us who are currently experiencing the symptoms of hormones going haywire—and twenty million more right behind us. Every eight minutes, an American woman turns fifty; within the next twenty-five years, more than fifty million American women will be over that mile marker.

Second, a major change has compelled me to write this book. Treatment options for women struggling through hormonal change—and its maladies—have changed drastically. When it comes to questions about hormones and hormone replacement, the entire medical community is in a midlife crisis!

If you aren't yet familiar with the tidal wave of startling research on hormone replacement for women that started to crash in on us all in the summer of 2002, I'm going to get you caught up. First, a study on estrogen-containing products was suddenly halted because it unveiled potentially serious side effects in postmenopausal women. Performed as part of the United States government-sponsored Women's Health Initiative (WHI), the study was stopped three years earlier than expected because of emerging evidence showing a small yet statistically significant increase in the risk of heart disease, breast cancer, stroke, and blood clots. Almost simultaneously, the National Institutes of Health released an international expert study that reported little to no benefits of HRT beyond treating hot flashes, vaginal dryness, and, in some cases, mood swings.

Most health practitioners were aware of the NIH report questioning HRT's effectiveness, but even I was taken by surprise with the WHI study's abrupt halt. The impact of these reports over the past few years is staggering. An estimated 6.5 million women have stopped taking hormones since the first report on HRT risks was released in 2002. Clients of mine who had previously sworn allegiance to their hormone prescriptions began tossing them out the window. I'm seeing sixty- and seventy-year-olds being hit with intense withdrawal symptoms from suddenly going off HRT, having more hot flashes than they did in their forties and fifties. And women just entering into the fray are at a loss of how to deal with their symptoms.

I'll discuss these studies in detail in chapter 7, but for now let me just say that women whose hormones are going haywire are in a state of confusion—and panic.

So *much* research has been released in the last few years, I felt it was time to update you on the results, further direct you in what to do *now*, and provide you with all the necessary tools for hormone balance—and total well-being—for life!

It's strange how often many women have approached me with their struggles of hormonal imbalance, yet when I point them toward *Take Charge of the Change* (the earlier edition of this book), they say, "Oh, thank God I'm not there yet." *Yet they are!* So I've not only revised and updated the contents, I've retitled the book as well. *When Your Hormones Go Haywire* is designed to meet the need of the woman thirty-something and beyond, showing how to take charge of the change *before*, *during*, and *beyond* the change.

Live Well, Live Blessed!
Pam

Part 1

THE
BEST PERIOD

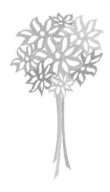

Life Cycles, Crashes, and Crossings

Whether you're in your late thirties, forties, or early fifties, you know that your body is behaving differently from what it once did. It *is* different, and not just because of the never-ceasing stress demands of life—career, family, too much to do, too little time to do it. Sure, those stresses show in occasional dark circles under our eyes, but there's more.

Now there are those unpredictable moods, the restless nights, roller-coaster energy levels, expanding waistlines, fuzzy thinking, heart palpitations, surprise tears, anxiety and paranoia, strange appetite cravings. Maybe you are still having periods, but they're not the same. They're shorter, longer, less painful, more painful, heavier, and lighter, and you can no longer set your clock by them. In fact, very little about your monthly cycle is the way it used to be. Or maybe it's regular as rain. You're on the pill, after all, so all these maladies couldn't possibly be related to your periods. Or could they?

Many women sail through their personal midlife crossing, noticing little different with their bodies except that periods have stopped and it's even harder to manage their weight. Others feel as though they've entered a storm from which they may never emerge, as though they've been caught in hurricane winds that threaten to blow away their emotional and physical health.

Many others, although thrilled to be "over" periods and raising children, will nonetheless find their body's reaction to this time of life to be a royal pain. Hot flashes, insomnia, those mood swings, and crying jags.

This note came from Kay:

> My weight hadn't changed but a few pounds, but my body sure didn't look the same. My entire shape has changed—when I see myself in the mirror, I can't believe it's my body, or that I'm not 4 months pregnant.
>
> And my body doesn't feel the same. I'm only forty-eight and my joints hurt—sometimes enough to wake me up at night. But the reality is, I'm waking up most nights anyway, and not easily getting back to sleep. Am I waking up a little hotter, sometimes sweating? Sometimes—but I'm surely not waking up in the morning rested nor replenished.
>
> I've had a physical and blood work and everything checks out. So I spend hours wondering if this is just what it feels like to be almost 50—or could it be my hormones?

Funny, I've been asked and asking that question since fifth grade when I had my first period. And here we are—thirty-something, forty-something, fifty-something—and still looking for answers. Are these feelings a sign that I'm sick, or stressed, or is it really *just my hormones*? As if that makes it tolerable somehow!

You would think we would have been better prepared for *this* period—something akin to being shown that "movie" in grade school or getting our "Kotex Starter Kit" (remember the sanitary belts?). Yet, most of us aren't any more prepared than we were then. It's come too early; we're confused and frustrated—and somewhat irritated with our bodies.

I surely know that I am, and I know that many of you are as well, based on the overwhelming pleas for help that come to my practice, seminars, and website. A good number of the questions come from women who have faithfully been living healthy lifestyles and are uncertain as to why their bodies are no longer responding in the same way. Why can't they get a good night's sleep anymore? Where did this five-pounds-through-the-tummy come from, and why won't it go away? They are desperate for direction and guidance in dealing with the changes they are being slammed with—and they want to know what to do now.

How now shall I eat? What are phytoestrogens; will they help or hurt? If I'm taking estrogen, should I avoid soy? What if I've had breast cancer? My physician says I need to gain weight to get my hormones in balance;

how do I do that without getting fat? Am I waking up in the middle of the night because my blood sugars are dropping? Should I be eating a bedtime snack? Should I be taking vitamin E? Can I do anything nutritionally to shrink fibroids? Is walking enough for exercise; should I be strength training? Is there anything I can do about my expanding waistline — and shrinking tolerance?

And, with the hormone controversies that have erupted in the last few years: *Should I go off my hormones? Cold turkey? And, if I'm not doing HRT, how do I prevent hot flashes — and osteoporosis? Are natural hormones better — or safer? Have you heard of black cohosh? Are anti-depressants a sign of surrender?*

Women in midlife are in a state of confusion — and panic.

We certainly aren't the first women in history to experience hormonal changes; after all, we watched our moms go through them. But they didn't talk much about it, and we sure didn't ask. We certainly *are* the first generation to knowledgeably question the way midlife has always been done and to choose to do it "our way," a new way — and a healthy one.

WE ARE *NOT* OUR MOTHERS

Regardless of how our mothers rode out their personal midlife storm, we are looking for a better way, certain that it must exist. Most of our moms lived through "The Change" silently, isolated from other women, quietly wondering if they were losing their minds along with their periods (even the word "menopause" was taboo in social and medical circles; hence the code word "The Change").

Many of us remember stormy moments with even the calmest of mothers — times when even June Cleaver-like moms went a bit schizoid. For some, those times may have resulted in much family pain and tragedy — my sister-in-law's mother took her life; another's went through a difficult divorce. For the lucky ones, our moms' "moments" were something to chuckle about — daily going on a treasure hunt for her missing keys, playing "period-math" to figure out why she woke up as the Wicked Witch of the West . . . or why she was crying at Johnson and Johnson commercials.

Our mothers' physicians rarely suggested HRT unless their symptoms were incapacitating. If it was prescribed, our moms simply did what they were told, even though they understood neither the risks nor reasons for such treatment. And they certainly had no idea that there was anything else they could do with their lifestyle to make a positive difference in their menopause experience.

A DIFFERENT DAY

Compare this scenario to Valerie, a forty-two-year-old boomer who has started noticing changes in her body — her energy, her weight, her moods, her sleep, her libido. She has gained eight pounds in three months without any change in her eating or exercise, and it has all gone to her abdomen. Feeling almost pregnant and definitely fatigued and frazzled, she goes to her doctor, hoping he will assure her that all is well, that it's only stress. Perhaps he will simply urge her to take that vacation she's been postponing. If only her health insurance would cover the cost of a Caribbean cruise!

Instead, he interrupts her island daydreams by prescribing a low-dose contraceptive pill that will give her a hormone boost, matter-of-factly informing her that she has entered the ranks of the perimenopausal. Her doctor explains that her body is starting to be affected by fluctuations in hormone levels in her bloodstream.

Menopausal? The word stuns her. *Am I really that old? Okay, he said "**peri**menopausal," but it sure sounds like the beginning of the end!*

Truly, more than simple fatigue has been plaguing her lately. She can't sleep, can't concentrate, suffers from migraines, feels bloated, and occasionally breaks out in sweats. She has been too busy to dwell on these symptoms; she has tossed the blame on the huge project she is working on. So maybe it's more. Maybe it's not just a matter of getting some needed time off now and then and exercising a little more.

Interestingly, Valerie doesn't fill that prescription for the pill; she isn't ready for hormone replacement, low dose or otherwise — certainly not now, with menopause possibly being years away. At the same time, she doesn't want to live with the symptoms she is experiencing. And that's what brings Valerie to me for coaching in taking charge of her health as naturally as possible. If HRT may ultimately be necessary, it is not going to be her first course of action. She determines that the perimenopausal diagnosis is just the wake-up call she needs to start taking care of her body—and soul—in full measure.

Valerie's goal? It's the same as my goal and, most likely, yours: feel well, look great, and live well. She wants to live as a whole woman—body, soul, and spirit—not as one torn apart at the seams. Valerie is ready to reclaim her joy and her purpose. It's the heart-cry of every woman between the age of thirty and fifty-five. (Forget that; it's the heart cry of every woman, regardless of age!) We are not ready to simply accept such problems as normal and be silent sufferers of "The Change" happening to us. Instead, we are ready to *take charge* of our own well-being in a whole new way—employing natural solutions for physical maladies, trading in emotional havoc for emotional stability, and receiving God's strength in our areas of weakness.

Here's a report from Kara, her "before and after" story, of sorts. The change she is experiencing after she has "taken charge of her change" by employing the Hormone Balancing Plan is in a word, amazing!

Before:	took approximately 4 powerful migraine pills each month for migraine headaches
Now:	months pass without needing to take even one
Before:	several days of feeling very emotional /depressed around the time of my period and ovulation; needing to take Prozac for a week during that time
Now:	minimal emotional change; have eliminated drugs
Before:	low energy, tired, no desire to keep up with my sons, ages 5, 9, 15
Now:	high energy, enthusiasm for life, enjoy activity with my family and friends
Before:	excessive use of caffeine, Nutrasweet, and sugar to get and keep me going
Now:	realize that those things kept me from going; stopped using them and changed to water, healthy foods, movement, sleep, and faith to get me going
Before:	70 pounds overweight
Now:	have lost 40 pounds, slowly, and know that more will come off!
Before:	considerable joint pain
Now:	considerably less pain
Before:	waking up several times a night
Now:	peaceful sleep

Before:	feeling foggy or fuzzy or headachy
Now:	feeling clear
Before:	**guilt** of how I was eating and how I was feeding my family; also guilt over the example I was setting; **fear** about my health and the future health of my family
Now:	**peace**

Thank you!! Thank you!! For helping me take charge of *my* change—balancing my hormones and reclaiming energy for life!

Perimenopause: The Midlife Crossing

In simplest terms, menopause is the final end to menstruation—medically defined as that point in time when our periods stop permanently. But of course, it is not a simple event; the biological changes are quite complex. Nor does menopause happen overnight. It's part of a longer life transition—this perimenopausal passage of some ten to fifteen years—during which the levels of key hormones that control our reproductive system change. The period approximately two years before and two years after the final menstrual period is clinically defined as perimenopause (meaning "around" or "near" menopause), but the name is often used to describe the entire premenopausal time.

We really have no way of knowing whether any given period is truly our last until a year has passed. But as menopause approaches, cycles become erratic, and months can go by without a period, only to show up once more. I've been waiting for months now for another, and although there have been warning signs that a whopper is coming, it hasn't happened—yet.

Most women will agree that stopping periods is not a bad thing, that the very *best* period in life is the *last* one! The average woman has approximately five hundred menstrual periods finally bringing her to the threshold of her menopause. But the absence of menstruation, which is the most obvious sign of menopause, is only one aspect of the transition. "The constant change of hormone levels during perimenopause can have a troubling effect on emotions," reports the American College of Obstetricians and Gynecologists. "Some women have mood swings, memory lapses, and poor concentration. Some say they cry for no reason. Some feel irritable or are depressed."

Well, my friend, this is an understatement.

TROUBLED WATERS?

Beyond our periods changing, most of the hormonal changes associated with perimenopause are well under way by the age of forty. If a woman is under significant stress at the same time (and who isn't?)—if she is overworked and underfueled on any level—her ability to keep up with the demands on her hormone production sites is even more compromised. The result may be an early and/or stormy midlife crossing, as she is slammed with her own individual combination of symptoms—from headaches to indigestion, hot flashes to bloating, depression to fuzzy thinking, lackluster libido to mood swings, mid-section weight gain to disrupted sleep. And it is no surprise that this torrent of physical symptoms can have a profound effect on her sense of spiritual well-being and her emotional demeanor.

Until the HRT scare of 2002, the typical approach for treating these symptoms was to prescribe something to soothe us and make us feel better. Have you noticed that we rarely ask ourselves (and certainly, doctors seldom ask), "What is out of balance that needs attention?" If we look to hormonal replacement for relief without addressing whole life issues, then even appropriate doses of hormones won't help much.

Have you ever considered that each menstrual period provides a snapshot of your place of balance—or imbalance. Consider how each one gives expression to your deepest needs and provides you the opportunity to take care of areas within your body and soul desperately crying out to be noticed.

How is your physical health and nutrition? *It shows during your period.* How are your stress levels and emotions? *It shows during your period.* What's happening in your relationships and career? *It shows during your period.* Is it well with your soul? *It shows during your period.*

At perimenopause, the body makes one final hormonally staged attempt to get us to deal with our issues of stress and self-care. If we've ignored those monthly snapshots up to now, the havoc we are experiencing may not allow us any longer to put our needs aside. Our body's response to the hormonal shifts is a reflection of how we care for ourselves today and how we have lived up to this point. Intolerable symptoms can become the opportunity to implement much needed change to make the next forty to fifty years the very *best* years. Now is the time to take stock and make sure that we are doing everything possible to retain, restore, or rebuild our health — and reclaim wholeness and connectedness. The very steps we take to remedy the midlife maladies of today lay the foundation for living great, looking great, and feeling great — for life.

MENOPAUSE: DESIGN OR DISEASE?

Other cultures have a greatly different attitude toward menopause than our own. In some cultures it is seen as a positive change — freedom from the need for contraception and from the ups and downs of the monthly period, and the arrival of a new status of "wise woman." Yet in our society, the change of life is seen as a kind of deficiency disease that emerges when we get to a certain age and our hormones decline.

That deficiency model of menopause dictates that if we add back these hormones, we would have a "cure" — or at least a management — for the disease. Diabetes, a disease caused by a specific hormone deficiency, is a good case in point. In diabetes, the hormone insulin is not present in sufficient amounts to maintain normal blood sugar levels, so all that is needed is for insulin to be supplied from outside and the imbalance is corrected.

But diabetes is an illness; menopause is not. All women will go through menopause; thankfully, we are not all going to get diabetes.

I believe that we were *created* for the change — God designed it as part of our natural life process — and perimenopause is a natural crossing through it. I don't believe that it's a dirty trick played on women, a life sentence, or a sickness to be tolerated.

Similar to puberty and pregnancy, there is a master plan and purpose genetically scripted into every cell of the female body to orchestrate and direct the transformation we call menopause. God's design includes natural and necessary body changes *for a reason*.

If you experience uncomfortable symptoms (like morning sickness and leg cramps in pregnancy, or mood swings and cramps in adolescence), how long they last and how intense they may be is dependent on a number of factors. In midlife, these include the type of menopause being experienced (natural or artificial—i.e., brought on by surgery or chemotherapy), our personal physical makeup, what else is going on in life, the ability of our bodies and souls to support us through this period of transition, and even our dieting history. The earlier you detect that things may be going awry and act to restore your body balance, the easier it will be to stay in that place of balance as you approach menopause. Even if your menopause is a decade or more away, how you treat yourself now will play a pivotal role in how you feel later.

The good news is that *symptoms*—whatever they may be for any one of us—are not what life is going to feel like from this day forward. We came through adolescence and maybe pregnancy, and we will come through this period too. The process can be a time of growth and preparation as we are being fashioned for a new life.

Like puberty, perimenopause may be a stormy shift in hormones, but in reverse—winding down rather than building up. With the exception of hot flashes, it's the mirror image of our teen years—externally and internally—and like that tumultuous time, the transition will end. Weight will stabilize, moods will even out, and thinking will clear. But rather than trying to navigate the tumultuous waters as an *in*experienced young girl, you can ride the waves as a woman. At the end, you will emerge ready and able to carry out your purpose and calling.

Most of us want a terrific life for our years ahead, one characterized by greater energy, vitality, and peace along with this renewed sense of purpose. We want to overcome the maladies of midlife—weight gain, fatigue, hot flashes, lost libido, and depression. The problem is that most women don't have a clue how to claim that abundant life or even where to begin, especially when things seem so out of balance now.

STARVING FOR ANSWERS

As shrouded in mystery as it may have been at one time, the midlife transition is receiving a lot of press in these baby-boomers-turning-forty-and-fifty days. It's here, it's reality, and like everything else in our lives, we are going to do it with gusto.

We are an information-hungry generation, so advice about hormonal change is available to satisfy every appetite, from every corner: books, magazine articles, health-care professionals, talk shows, friends, family, the internet.

Sometimes this can be too much of a good thing. If you are deciding how to handle hot flashes, for example, you may be bombarded with conflicting suggestions.

- Your mom tells you to tough it out; she did.
- Your friend is getting acupuncture and thinks you should too.
- Your sister has become a poster child for the local herb shop and wants you to do exactly what she's doing.
- One book advises Hormone Replacement Therapy to protect against osteoporosis, yet a TV doctor emphatically advises against HRT because of breast cancer risk.
- Your neighbor has had miraculous success using natural progesterone.
- Your gynecologist doesn't agree that progesterone would be right for you, especially in the form of a "worthless yam cream," as she calls it.

So how do you begin to sort out all this advice and figure out what's right for *you*? We are being hit from all sides by the claims, counterclaims, and controversy about estrogen or progesterone replacement. We worry about taking hormones, and we worry about *not* taking them and possibly shortchanging ourselves, now or later in life.

Take a deep breath—and read on. This book is written to give you new perspective on your needs and practical guidance on how you can best meet them—for reclaiming your energy, fitness, and vitality in the physical realm, and for entering a new place of peace and joy emotionally and spiritually.

Cutting-edge research is now available to explain better what happens when hormones go awry, why you feel good when your hormones are in sync, and why you feel horrible when they aren't. You will soon learn what is happening when your delicate balance of body chemistries gets tipped, impacting metabolism, moods, memory, energy, sex drive, fluid balance, and temperature regulation.

I want you to know this: Whether or not you choose to take supplemental hormones for a short time, there are additional ways to relieve the symptoms of hormonal imbalance through nutrition, exercise, and lifestyle enhancements, which are virtually risk free. These natural solutions to midlife maladies stand on their own or can work together with a spritz of HRT, if necessary. This is the essence of true complementary medicine—using lifestyle as preventative medicine and making appropriate adjustments to stabilize the body processes—so that if further medication or treatment is required, it is in reduced amounts.

When your hormones go haywire, you can *take charge* of your health, not so that you can simply "ride out the storm" but so that you can live life to the full—fully living in God's design and unique purpose for you.

Here's a note from Jodie, who has done just that:

> I was feeling the typical perimenopausal symptoms—foggy brain, unexplained weight gain, irregular periods, migraine headaches, etc.—when I gave the Hormone Balance Plan a try. I never in my life believed that so many symptoms could be associated with hormone imbalance and on the flip side never had such a complete turn around on so many ailments. I'm hooked on healthy eating and so grateful. I don't have the foggy brain and don't have to search for words when I'm in conversation. My weight is decreasing as I've found energy to exercise. My irregular periods aren't so bothersome since I'm in control now. And I haven't had a migraine since the first two weeks on the plan. I'm glad this worked instead of having to go through what so many of my friends went through to alleviate perimenopausal symptoms. They've been on so many drugs!

Hormones: Terrorists
or Peacekeepers?

Whether it's a period, menopause, stress, a hysterectomy, or plain old heredity, women have felt vulnerable to hormonal hurricanes for years, long before midlife.

We've called "raging" hormones PMS (premenstrual syndrome); jokes about it abound, as does the surrounding misery. Perimenopausal hormonal change can bring PMS to an art form.

For some women, the hormonal shifts that produce those same physical and emotional symptoms commonly associated with PMS—mood swings, fatigue, and bloating—escalate as they get into their late thirties. Then the classic menopausal symptoms such as hot flashes and insomnia begin during perimenopause. And symptoms can develop at a relatively young age, so that PMS and menopause often converge into "The Perfect Storm." If you've ever seen the movie, you understand the helplessness and terror of being tossed to and fro by waves of great magnitude.

Without an exhaustive biology lesson, some basic discussion of the science of hormones is important to fully understand how they impact your well-being, both body and soul. The brain's site of hormone production is the same as that for metabolism control, fluid balance, blood sugar regulation, and thyroid function; all of these are impacted by the slightest change in brain chemicals. And, like Humpty Dumpty, they can all come tumbling down at once, seemingly to "never be put back together again."

JUST THE BASICS

With all the life struggle associated with hormones, it's easy to forget the vital truth: Female hormones are not the enemy! They are not designed to make us sick or miserable; rather, they are meant to keep us well! Our hormones are for more than childbearing alone; they enhance our physical, emotional, and mental well-being.

Because of this, we begin life fully equipped to produce all the hormones we will ever need throughout life. Long after reproduction is no longer feasible, there continue to be vital roles for the so-called reproductive hormones—jobs that have nothing to do with making babies. And there is an ongoing production of these hormones to help our bodies perform phenomenal functions, protect us from premature aging and disease, and serve to nourish our hair, skin, bones, heart, and brain.

Hormones are simply chemicals, designed by God for important purposes and produced by our endocrine glands. The two hormones most familiar to women are estrogen and progesterone, but there are many more, such as testosterone. They all have an intimate relationship with other chemicals produced by our brains—that is, with neurotransmitters such as serotonin, dopamine, and norepinephrine. This interplay—especially between your hormones and serotonin—impacts how you feel, look, and think. It can transform battle zones into safe havens and peaceful living into war.

ESTROGEN: OUR CHANGING FRIEND

Estrogen is the key hormone responsible for the transition from childhood to womanhood. It causes our breasts to develop and produces our feminine shape. It also causes the lining of the uterus to thicken each month in anticipation of receiving a fertilized egg. Estrogen not only serves in the regulation of the menstrual cycle, but it also acts as a mild antidepressant and greatly enhances a woman's sense of well-being. When estrogen is not at proper levels in the body, memory, mood, and sex drive all suffer—which explains the many changes associated with menopause as estrogen production begins to dramatically change. Before this, there is a natural ebb and flow to hormones, as estrogen levels peak in the first two weeks of the menstrual cycle—about twelve days in—and decrease during the last two weeks after ovulation.

The peak of estrogen production stimulates ovulation, and the ovary begins to produce progesterone to help the uterus prepare for the fertilized egg. Progesterone levels further increase when the estrogen levels begin to decrease and stay high over the last two weeks of the cycle. When fertilization does not take place, there is a release of the thickened lining of the uterus (the period) and a decrease in the production of both hormones, which alerts the body to the need to get the cycle started again. And so it goes, month after month, generally for more than thirty years. With the exception of pregnancy or extreme stress, the cycle is rarely broken.

Generally, two to ten years before menopause, ovulation becomes less likely each month because the ovaries simply begin to run out of eggs. With fewer and fewer eggs, the production of estrogen and the cyclic release of progesterone become erratic and less ample.

As the ovaries become less responsive, there is a rising level of FSH, the follicle-stimulating hormone produced in the brain. Yet its demand outplays the ovaries' supply; too little estrogen is produced, or surges in estrogen result and the delicate balance between progesterone and estrogen levels can go awry. Without adequate levels of estrogen, the lining of the uterus doesn't thicken in preparation for a baby. Or,

Predicting your Last Period

The average woman has her last period around her fifty-first birthday. That doesn't mean, however, that most women experience menopause when they are fifty-one, only that half of all women stop menstruating before they turn fifty-one and half stop menstruating afterward. In the U.S., the statistics for the age women experience natural menopause (as compared to that brought on by surgery or other procedures) break down like this: 10% by age 38, 30% by age 44, 50% by age 49, 90% by age 54, and 100% by age 58.

There's no established correlation between the age at which you start your period and the age you reach menopause, or between menopause and your race, height, number of children you have, or whether or not you took birth control pills or ever were pregnant — although all of these factors are being studied to explain why this generation of American women seem to be entering perimenopause at younger ages than previous ones. There may be some correlation with smoking as well as the age your mother was when she reached menopause.

if too much estrogen is produced but too little progesterone, the lining becomes thick and heavy, resulting in flood-like periods, and the woman is robbed of progesterone's tranquilizing, sleep-enhancing properties.

As the calendar continues to turn, ovulation becomes more and more erratic — irregular, at unexpected times of the month, or not at all some months. Finally, no ovulation occurs — ever again — and the menstruation cycle stops. This is menopause.

A CHANGE IN PRODUCTION

Contrary to popular belief, the ovaries don't entirely shut down when you stop having menstrual cycles. They don't shrivel up and die after menopause; they only slow down production and change their product line.

The ovary is a very complex gland with a multitude of functions. The thin outer layer (the ovarian theca) produces eggs; that layer becomes increasingly nonfunctional as you move out of the childbearing years. However, the inner layer (the ovarian stroma) is capable of producing all of the steroid hormones (estrogen, progesterone, testosterone, and more), and it functions throughout your life. During perimenopause, the stroma picks up its production of estrogen, but in a weaker form (which gets converted to a stronger estrogen) in smaller quantities, and without ovulation.

In addition, the adrenal glands (which sit atop the kidneys) produce this same hormone, which is used alongside the ovaries' diminishing supply, and both make their way to the fat cells, where it is converted to a stronger type of estrogen called estrone. Hence, body fat becomes the main manufacturing site for midlife estrogen.

> **Did You Know?**
>
> Body fat taking over as the main manufacturing site for midlife estrogen is why estrogen levels are higher than normal in overweight midlifers and why extra weight gives some protection from pre- and post-menopausal symptoms. The extra estrogen produced from the fat cells balances the estrogen decline from the ovaries. Therefore, the midlife body is on a mission to build bigger and better fat cells to be the new production factories for new forms of estrogen.

Please know that an expanding waistline at perimenopause is not just about what you are eating, the exercise you do or don't do, or the fact that you are feeling the effects of post-forty metabolic slow-down. Your body is using all of these factors to accomplish one of its more important life moves: transferring your hormone production to new sites. The most efficient estrogen production comes from abdominal fat cells—which is why even women who have never struggled with that spot suddenly start to get a tummy.

It's not a trick, it's all part of your Intelligent Design. Without a few pounds of added fat, your hormone supply will be at a serious deficit, and the symptoms of hormonal imbalance will be greatly exaggerated. A little more midsection weight, and the symptoms will be much milder. (*Finally*, a reason for twenty-first-century women to rejoice at a few extra pounds on the scale!) We'll talk more about this later (see chapter 16), and be encouraged: I will give you specific strategies to crack the midlife fat cell code.

In addition to the fat cells taking on estrogen production, we also begin to produce progesterone and testosterone at other sites, such as the skin and the brain. Our body is more than willing to increase the output from these other sites as the need arises at midlife. Hormone receptors are found in almost every organ of our bodies, and our bodies are even designed with the ability to convert one type of hormone into another.

Hormones in Action

FSH (follicle stimulating hormone) and **LH (luteinizing hormone)**, produced in the pituitary gland in the brain. They stimulate the rise of estrogen and progesterone during the monthly menstrual cycle.

Estrogen, produced primarily in the ovaries before menopause and primarily in body fat afterwards. Estrogen is the class of hormones; the body actually makes many types. Here are the three main ones: estradiol (produced by fertile ovaries), estrone (produced from the conversion of estradiol in the fat cells), and estriol (the weakest form, produced from the conversion of estrone).

Progesterone, produced primarily in the ovaries. It works with estrogen to prepare the lining of the uterus for implantation and growth of a baby and works with brain chemicals to bring a sense of calm into life.

Estrogen can be converted into testosterone; progesterone can be converted into estrogen.

All of this hormone production—albeit in different sites, from different sources—is why the term Hormone Replacement Therapy is a misnomer. It's more accurately called hormone *addition* therapy, picking up the slack and helping the body along through the transition process.

THE DELICATE BALANCE

The coordinated movement of the manufacture and dispersal of hormones in a woman's body is like an orchestra, where all the instruments need to play together to achieve balance and harmony. It doesn't take much to throw the hormonal symphony into havoc. As vital as estrogen is to our brains and bodies, it's the delicate interplay between estrogen and progesterone that impacts our overall well-being during the perimenopausal masterpiece. Progesterone levels are apt to fall dramatically—often long before there are any changes in estrogen or testosterone levels—and this is of major significance to our overall well-being. If the progesterone is too low, other hormones may miss their cues and drop notes. If the estrogen is too high, it may drown out the progesterone.

When estrogen levels surge or progesterone levels fall short of the normal range, the imbalance can result in a myriad of premenstrual mood changes: anxiety, depression, irritability, anger, tearfulness, and/or mental fuzziness. Our bodies are very sensitive to hormonal balance, and even small hormone fluctuations can wreak havoc—not just during menopause but on a monthly basis throughout menstruation. Nor is the havoc just a day or two before our menstrual cycle. Many of us experience lethargy, moodiness, sleeplessness, and fatigue from ovulation through the end of our period. We barely get a breath of energy before the symptoms begin again. In perimenopause, it can seem like a thirty-day battle that strikes *every* thirty days.

Every woman experiences perimenopause differently. Some have virtually no symptoms; others have every one in the book. Because the range of symptoms is so diverse, many women don't make the connection with hormonal imbalance and so they suffer in silence, blame it on stress, or move from one specialist to another looking for cures. If you are experiencing any of the following, ask your gynecologist if he or she thinks you may be in perimenopause:

- irregular periods
- increasing PMS symptoms—bloating, cramps, breast tenderness
- hot flashes and/or night sweats
- insomnia and fatigue
- heart palpitations
- mood swings, irritability, and/or paranoia
- migraine headaches
- memory problems
- fuzzy thinking or inability to concentrate
- dry, itchy, irritated skin
- dry, dull, or thinning hair
- brittle nails
- weight gain, especially around the middle
- vaginal dryness, itchiness, or recurring infections
- pain with intercourse
- loss of interest in sex
- urinary tract infection
- frequent urination or stress incontinence
- achy joints
- indigestion, burping, and gas
- increased irritable bowel syndrome

As natural of a process as perimenopause may be, it's a force to be reckoned with, especially when the body's hormonal harmony goes awry. However, although some symptoms are common to this time of life, *extreme* symptoms aren't normal and are not a "given." Yet, as many as 10 to 15 percent of women are immobilized by them.

TESTING IT OUT:
HOW DO I KNOW IT'S MY HORMONES?

Unfortunately, simply measuring blood levels of estrogen or progesterone is not really useful for determining your menopausal status because the levels in the blood fluctuate widely and wildly. There is also a question about just how important it is to know the exact levels of hormones circulating in the body at any given time, because certain levels don't necessarily add up to certain symptoms. Yet, along with charting physical, emotional, and mental symptoms on paper, hormone testing can often be useful for getting a clearer picture for appropriate treatment. I particularly suggest laboratory tests when HRT appears to be the only answer for symptom relief, to identify the right "brew."

A more accurate test than measuring blood levels of estrogen or progesterone is to measure the blood level of FSH, the hormone that stimulates ovulation. FSH levels tend to rise dramatically around menopause as a direct result of decreased levels of estrogen, as much as fifteen times higher than they were earlier. An FSH level over twenty reflects a perimenopausal state; over forty reveals a low estrogen level and probably menopause. (Interestingly enough, FSH surges are thought to be the culprit behind hot flashes.)

However, during perimenopause, even FSH levels can fluctuate a great deal, so there is a growing body of health specialists who do not put their faith in those levels either. Depending on when you're tested, you will get different readings. Blood tests for levels of FSH can tell you how much FSH you're producing at the moment, but it can't tell you how much you were producing five years ago or how much you'll be producing in the next half hour.

Because of this, many health care providers have turned to saliva testing as a more accurate read on the "free hormone" activity in the body. Unfortunately, even these tests have not been borne out in research as of yet and have also been shown to give false reads on hormone status.

The most important test is one you give yourself—a self-assessment of your symptoms and your lifestyle of self-care. You will find a Food-Feelings-and-Findings Journal (see p. 137); it will guide you on the path of discovery as you come to understand how you really feel and how you care for yourself, day by day. This book was designed to give you both a starting place and a destination: *hormone balance*.

A HORMONE OF ANOTHER KIND: THYROID

It may be perimenopause, but what is most frequently misdiagnosed as menopause is hyperthyroidism. That's because the symptoms, which can include flushing, sweating, heat intolerance, heart palpitations, and sleeplessness, can easily be confused with those of menopause.

In hyperthyroidism, the thyroid produces excess amounts of thyroid hormone, thyroxine, which overstimulates organs and speeds up many of the body's functions. If left untreated, an overactive thyroid can cause a loss of bone mineral density, which, over time, can lead to osteoporosis. Hyperthyroidism can also result in an irregular heartbeat, which can lead to stroke or heart failure.

Unintended weight loss almost always accompanies an overactive thyroid. So if you're losing weight while not trying to, your heart frequently beats rapidly, or you're always hot even when people around you are cold, don't just blame menopause. There's a difference between the intermittent flushing and sweating associated with perimenopause and just being hot and sweating all the time.

A simple blood test called a TSH (thyroid-stimulating hormone) test will diagnose hyperthyroidism. (It is more accurate than older tests.) TSH, which is made by the pituitary gland, regulates the amount of thyroid hormone that is released into the blood. When the thyroid gland produces too much thyroid hormone, the pituitary compensates by pumping out less TSH. So a TSH level below normal could be a warning sign.

I typically see more issues with *hypo*thyroidism than *hyper-*. Women between the ages of thirty and fifty are most typically affected with hypothyroidism, and it's estimated that 10 percent of women age forty and older go undiagnosed. That's one reason that the American Association of Clinical Endocrinologists recommends that all women over the age of forty have a TSH screening test. With hypothyroidism, the TSH will be abnormally high because of the unresponsive thyroid gland forcing more and more of the stimulating hormone to be produced.

Symptoms of an underactive thyroid can also be easily mistaken for signs of menopause: heavy menstrual bleeding, fatigue, painful joints, mood swings, and weight gain. Don't let your doctor dismiss these types of symptoms with "What do you expect at your age?" Ask for a TSH test. That way, you can avoid being given a prescription for estrogen replacement therapy when you really need to be treated for thyroid deficiency.

I'M STILL HAVING PERIODS— AND THEY AREN'T PRETTY!

When a woman is going through the hormonal changes of perimenopause, just about any kind of uterine bleeding is possible, ranging from periods that become very light and short to periods that space out to every three months or more. Some women have absolutely no change in their cycle; their perimenopausal symptoms are expressed in sleep disturbances, hot flashes, and the like. Some women have bleeding patterns that are so erratic that they don't seem like periods at all.

Irregular menstrual periods, one of the most common and predictable signs of menopause, most often occur because of the erratic levels of estrogen and progesterone and less frequent ovulation.

Every woman has a unique pattern to her periods and knows what's normal for her. But as you've already read, when approaching menopause, what's normal can seem to take on a whole new definition.

It is certainly expected that perimenopausal periods will differ from your usual pattern. But if something isn't familiar to you and represents a dramatic change, you need

Symptoms Checklist

Hyperthyroidism	Hypothyroidism
unexplained weight loss	unexplained weight gain
rapid heartbeat	heavy menstrual bleeding
hot and sweating	fatigue
	dry skin
	painful joints
	mood swings

to see a health provider to check it out. Menstrual changes that are considered abnormal and need to be checked out include:

- periods that are very heavy and gushing, or bleeding with clots
- periods that last more than seven days, or two or more days longer than usual
- spotting between periods
- bleeding after intercourse
- repeatedly fewer than twenty-one days between periods

Frequently these symptoms are left unquestioned and untreated for an inordinate amount of time. The troubling fact is that they could signal complications; getting the right diagnosis is crucial. Your doctor will want to know what triggers the bleeding and what makes it stop, will run tests to determine the cause of the abnormal bleeding, and will assess whether the blood loss is adversely affecting your iron levels.

Keeping a diary to track changes in your menstrual pattern is a good idea, so you can see when and where changes occur and share them with your physician. Taking a moment to record your lifetime menstrual history will be helpful to you both. Amazing realizations can come through even a short reflection on your life as it relates to your periods.

LIFE AS A PERIOD—
A PERFECT DEFINITION FOR *PERIOD*

I love Webster's definition 3.b. for period: end, stop. Amen to that! When women have been asked the question, "If you had a choice, would you rather say 'Yes' or 'No' to menopause?" the overwhelming majority answer "Yes!" To choose against menopause would be a choice for periods, PMS, cramps, Tampax, pads, bloating, contraception, or childbearing for the rest of our lives. Stopping periods is generally not our collective struggle, although something feels strangely amiss when that monthly rhythm is no longer there.

Regardless, I'm ready to be over periods—and maybe you are too. One of my clients *definitely* is! She wrote this as a proclamation of freedom:

Does it seem like much of your life has been staged around your period? It sure does for me. Desperately wanting it to come, to get it over with before the beach party, or prom, or finals—or my wedding day. I would plead with my body, just START! I knew I would feel better and less bloated and edgy, if I could just START!

I was always frightened when my period didn't come; I was relieved when it did, and usually angry and puzzled that it always did finally start on the first day of vacation, the day I had to give a major presentation, or anytime I wanted and needed to be at my best. Instead, thanks to my period, I would feel and look my worst.

So, enough! I'm ready to not have to wonder, every month, if I'm pregnant. I'm ready to be free from feeling hostage to PMS symptoms. I'm really, really ready for this change. A hot flash or two is a small price to pay.

If Eve was cursed with periods, menopause is indeed the blessing!

THE STRESS CONNECTION

Whether menopause is a blessing or a curse to you, hormones running amuck and affecting your very quality of life are definitely *not* the way menstruation should end and the rest of your life begin. Know this: Raging, wildly fluctuating hormones are not a given in perimenopause! When extreme symptoms of hormonal imbalance occur, it's the result of the sum of hormone levels, brain chemistry, and personal life situations.

Interestingly, although perimenopausal hormone levels tend to fluctuate widely in all women, there's no rhyme or reason for exactly why some of us experience a stormier crossing. Trying to explain it or predict it can be like trying to explain or forecast the weather. Sometimes the analysis itself is immobilizing! It's far more productive to deal with what you are being dealt than to try to identify the why behind it.

However, there are other times that the road to "why" leads right back to that same old tired issue: negative, unprocessed stress. And to really deal with the hormonal imbalance, you first have to identify—and defuse—the stress connection.

STRESS: THE GOOD, THE BAD, AND THE UGLY

Stress is not always a bad thing, for it keeps us on our toes, alerts us to danger, and prepares us for challenge; it is essential to life. Yet, unprocessed stress can also make us frazzled or even sick. It can make us overweight and keep us that way because of its impact on metabolism and fat storage.

But did you know it also creates hormonal imbalance? It does! Stress affects the brain and all of its functions, including hormone and serotonin production, in addition to metabolic rate. We know that stress affects fertility because of the impact of stress hormones on the hypothalamus gland, which produces the reproductive hormones. And we know that stress can so affect the hormone production site of the brain that severe levels can even shut down menstruation.

With this knowledge, it's no surprise that stress is almost always involved when hormones go haywire and is most often the root of exaggerated perimenopausal maladies. Researchers theorize that the most disabling symptoms strike women who combine imbalanced lifestyles and stress demands with a midlife body that has a unique mix of physical predispositions.

So you're stressed to the max, and now you read that the stress is why you are also a hormonal mess. More stress. And stress begets stress. The resulting hormonal imbalance can result in a more intensive stress response, moodiness, depression, mental fuzziness, sleep deprivation, fatigue, hot flashes, and headaches. Actually, if you hold a list of the common symptoms of stress up to a list of the common symptoms of hormonal havoc, they look one and the same.

But let's face it: Life in this twenty-first century *is* stressful for us all! There is a frenzy to our lives that certainly contributes—if not being causal—to hormone imbalance. A majority of women, especially those thirty to fifty, report feeling more demands at home, and almost half say they are not as physically fit as they were even five years ago. The older we get, the more responsibilities we seem to have, and all too often that means we don't find the time to take care of ourselves.

As we approach age forty, the accrued stresses of a lifetime, declining metabolism, and the inevitable onset of perimenopause begin to take their toll on us. Our lives are especially frazzled at this age as we juggle various aspects of our lives (teenagers, spouse, career, aging parents, household matters, church, and friends), and hormones, including stress hormones, are beginning to flood our body somewhat unpredictably. Our desire to be good daughters, good mothers, good wives, good friends, and purposeful in life runs headlong into the increasingly urgent need to take care of ourselves and the needs of our souls. The resulting competition between the conflicting desires and demands can wreak havoc with our health.

Whether or not this is the whole story, hormonal imbalance certainly hits hard at women who are already struggling to balance family and work, who forget to take care of themselves, and who aren't getting the support or fueling they need on any level. For them, there is no eye in this life hurricane.

But there *is* help available — for every woman, in every arena of life. We can reclaim our peace and be well and energized — body, soul, and spirit.

Keep reading!

DISTRESS

When a threatening event takes place, our bodies are miraculously crafted to swing into action. When the body reads a situation as life threatening, it triggers a "fight or flight" response. When triggered into the stress reaction, the body initiates a primal response to save your life. The primary messengers of the stress response are hormones called norepinephrine and epinephrine, which are often referred to together as adrenaline. They are produced in the brain and the adrenal glands.

Every time adrenaline levels go up, levels of that other adrenal hormone, cortisol, also go up. Together, these biochemicals activate the body to help us escape danger and live. Within seconds, the body is in high alert — a state of readiness. We are tingling, anxious. Our pupils dilate, blood pressure and sugars rise, thinking improves, the heart starts pumping more quickly. Breathing is faster; we are alert, focused, and energetic — ready and able to leap tall buildings in a single bound! These hormones are responsible for the supernatural strength that rises up to allow a ninety-eight-pound fourteen-year-old girl to pick up a couch and throw it out a window in order to save herself and her baby sister from a fire. Or a mother to pick up a car to save a trapped infant. What amazing power can come through our miraculous body design!

After the initial mental stress-shock, the body returns to its "normal" state, and the hormones that have flooded the muscles and tissues with these important survival messages gradually leave the blood stream. However, cortisol lingers in the system and is designed to help bring everything back into balance, telling the body that all is well and that the danger has passed.

But what happens when stress comes in waves, again and again, and is never resolved? If the stress hormones continue to wash through the system at high levels, never leaving the body? The stress takes on a life of its own, and you get stuck in the stress response. How easily that happens in today's world with the reality of the kinds of stresses that we endure every day!

In modern society we can no longer run from or fight our stresses; we have substituted mental and emotional stresses for physical ones. But our primal stress response is wired for some sort of physical response—one that just doesn't come in present day "dangers": complexities of our technical society, bombardment with disturbing news of global proportions, traffic woes, misbehaving kids, bosses and spouses, aging parents, unrelenting schedules and deadlines, aging bodies, and the like. They aren't the physical threats our ancestors faced, yet they are stresses nonetheless.

Not one single common stressor of today requires a physical response that provides a stress release. Rather, the stress is experienced from our heart up to our brain. Add the decline of estrogen and progesterone levels to the mix, and midlife can be a giant roller coaster ride—and not a fun one!

A WILD RIDE

Estrogen and stress hormones are closely associated, like cousins. Actually, stress hormones determine how well we cope with all of the hormonal milestones in our lives. When we begin to menstruate, stress hormones impact our mood, the severity of PMS and cramping, as well as cravings and appetite. During pregnancy, the stress hormones affect nausea, weight gain, and our tendency toward postpartum depression.

As women approach menopause and estrogen and progesterone levels become more erratic, waxing and waning, the stress hormones ride the same wild ride, impacting the entire body and brain function. In addition, the body begins to secrete higher levels of testosterone. Testosterone is a potent stimulator of intra-abdominal fat deposition and contributes to facial hair growth and mood changes.

The adrenal glands become overstimulated and exhausted, which results in an impairment of the cells' ability to metabolize fatty acids. This in turn results in a heightened susceptibility to weight gain as the body tends to break down muscle and replace it with stored fat and excess fluid. In addition, surges of cortisol stimulate an excess production of insulin, which affects everything from blood sugar regulation to even more fat storage.

And it doesn't end there. Increased cortisol in the bloodstream blocks progesterone from its receptors, impairing progesterone activity; it also interferes with estrogen production and prevents release of serotonin, the good news messenger for the body. With the decreased production of calming progesterone, life begins to "feel" even more stressful, hence begetting a stronger stress response and more hormone shifts. When these stress hormones and progesterone compete, the stress hormones win out—and they are not a good substitution; trading progesterone's calming action for cortisol's anxiety, shakiness, and headaches is no picnic. The result is that women who are chronically stressed also tend toward an even stronger hormonal imbalance between estrogen, progesterone, and testosterone.

When our hormone levels are fluctuating, our stress level can both influence and be a by-product of these chemical changes. Low progesterone and serotonin may produce anxious feelings, and our bodies try to mediate the effects of stress by pouring out more adrenaline and cortisol. High cortisol levels impact blood sugar levels, causing a much wider and wilder sensitivity. Blood sugar crashes stimulate the release of even more adrenaline, which in turn stimulates the release of cortisol, which in turn causes even more blood sugar fluctuations. It's just one of many downward spirals of ill health—but not an irreversible one.

Continuing in the same stressful situation with the same stress response virtually guarantees that our hormones will stay unbalanced. The longer we are overtaken by the negative, the more out of whack our hormones become and the more turmoil we stay in physically.

LEARN TO RIDE THE WAVE OF STRESS

Feeling overwhelmed just reading about the hormonal havoc working behind the scenes in your life? Ready to close this book in dismay, thinking there is no way out? I have good news for you. Simply by learning these biological facts, you are already on your way to discovering the power you have to make some life-altering choices.

Understanding how stress affects every single hormone and cell in your body and knowing how to defuse it gives you access to the most powerful and empowering health-creating secret on earth. The secret is this: The power is available to you to uncover a life of joy, abundance, and health, or to keep that freedom cloaked in a life filled with stress, fatigue, and disease. Wondrously and by design, the choice is yours.

To defuse stress does not mean walking away from all the things that cause it; rather, it means mounting a defensive and offensive strategy that enables you to ride the waves of stress rather than being capsized by them. It is possible—*without* quitting your job or marriage or putting your kids up for adoption! You have already begun to understand some of the building blocks you'll be using to bring a healthier structure to your life. One more chapter to explore some essentials, and you'll be prepared to put part 2 of this book to work for you.

Remember: You are not alone; God created you for this time, and he will guide you through it.

It's Not All in Your Mind, but It Is in Your Brain

Jenny, a forty-year-old client, came for coaching because of an everyday fatigue that was becoming more difficult to live with—a general loss of enthusiasm about life and living, resulting in a malaise that she couldn't shake. She wasn't sleeping well; she was waking up several times a night wet with sweat. She had gained weight and couldn't get focused on a plan to lose it. "Is it my age? Is it just that I'm a working mom? Are life demands too much to handle? Is it PMS?" She was having very regular periods, so she was certain she was too young for menopause.

As Jenny and I reviewed her day-to-day life, oh-too-familiar patterns began to emerge. The mother of a seven- and a two-year-old, she was married and worked fifty to sixty hours a week, many of them traveling. The demands of her work were considerable, and she found herself continually torn between work and the duties of being a wife and mom, with little or no time for herself.

We looked at the potential causes of her fatigue and burnout. Was she getting restful sleep? Was she eating energizing foods in a nourishing way? Any exercise? How was her help and support with the kids? Did she do anything to unwind from work—and home? She shrugged and sighed, "You've got to be kidding! Who has time?"

Jenny is a perfect example of a "lady boomer" with an extremely busy lifestyle—very smart and knowledgeable about nutrition, rest, and exercise but unable to establish a positive routine for herself. And her hormones were paying the price for her stress.

As with Jenny, one of the most common complaints of perimenopause is feeling tired and sluggish much of the time. Rather suddenly, or so it seems, women find they lack the energy to be the patient moms, supportive partners, or fun-loving friends and coworkers they would like to be. Although they know that exercise will help revive them, they rarely have the time, motivation, or energy.

Difficulty concentrating is another telltale sign, especially in women forty and older. Trouble focusing on tasks, absorbing complex information, and remembering names can be a source of embarrassment. Then comes the overeating and weight gain. Most women have little trouble controlling their appetite in the morning—they aren't hungry. Many can't even face food early in the day. But sometime in the afternoon, they begin to snack.

Because of the intricate interplay between hormones and the neurotransmitters of the brain, being caught in a hormone hurricane can bring destructive winds into our life picture, threatening to capsize us and take our loved ones down too. Proper nutrition, exercise, sleep—even exposure to sunlight—can be tremendous stabilizers, yet, if at a deficit, can fuel the hormonal hurricane. Sedentary women under stress, who skip meals and go long hours without balanced eating, will not weather the storm without taking a beating. Yet the storm's fury takes them by surprise—*because these habits are not new.* But here is your news flash, ladies: Your body's perimenopausal response *is* new—and very different.

> **Did You Know?**
>
> A craving for sweets and starches is one of the defining characteristics of hormonal imbalance. And because the body is on a mission to make bigger fat cells, every extra morsel goes to that means.

MORE THAN HORMONES

It's important to know that hormones such as estrogen and progesterone are just a *part* of our body symphony's amazing performance. It takes specific combinations of vitamins, minerals, enzymes, fatty acids, and energy to help the brain conduct the hormonal orchestra and to help the cells carry out the hormones' messages.

After years of working with women to get relief for PMS, I know that the escalation of symptoms around it is often an internal guidance system trying to get you to pay attention to the adjustments you need to make in life. I also know that these needed adjustments become particularly urgent during perimenopause. At midlife, the hormonal madness that was present only for a few days each month during most of the reproductive years now gets stuck in the "on" position for weeks or months at a time.

But hormonal madness need not continue. Whether you are reeling from PMS days or from perimenopausal years, a correct nutrition and lifestyle strategy can help you not only gain hormonal balance and reduce symptoms of hormonal imbalance today, but it will also protect you against tomorrow's risk of osteoporosis, heart disease, and cancer.

If you are suffering from hormonal imbalance, there are specific causes and specific solutions. With some personal sleuthing and creativity and a willingness to keep track of what works and what doesn't, hormonal imbalance can usually be brought *into* balance within a few months.

THE BRAIN ON HORMONES

Because God designed the brain as the prime spot for promoting hormonal balance, many of the strategies for reducing and/or eliminating symptoms simply come down to stabilizing brain chemistries. The first and vital step in stabilizing hormones and defusing stress response is learning to feed the brain to equalize hormone production and live in ways that promote positive serotonin and other neurotransmitter interplay.

You are about to discover that such change is far more manageable than you have imagined. But before we get started, let's better understand the physical design of your brain.

The hypothalamus, the body's control center in the brain, regulates the production of all the hormones and is in turn regulated by them. It has receptors not only for progesterone, estrogen, and androgens (such as DHEA and testosterone) but also for neurotransmitters (such as norepinephrine, dopamine, and sero-tonin) that work to set one's mood and that are in turn affected by our thoughts, beliefs, diet, and environment.

This control center, your hypothalamus, is affected by external as well as internal factors. It is the hypothalamus that is battered by the stress chemicals, causing the metabolism, blood sugars, fluid balance, and hormone production to go awry in times of intense stress. Little wonder that the symptoms of hormonal imbalance are metabolic slowdowns; fluctuations in blood sugar that result in irritability, fatigue, and increased appetite; and fluid retention and bloating.

Even something as "natural" as food cravings are controlled by the delicate balance of hormones and their action on your neu-rotransmitters, which is why it's so common to experience an extreme desire for chocolate or potato chips around the time of your period. But, as you will soon learn, you don't have to be con-trolled by such swings in your brain chemistry. It may be common, but it's not normal, and you need not fall victim to it. You will come to understand that you were created with a better plan in mind—a plan for peace, not war.

SEROTONIN: THE MESSENGER OF PEACE

One of the neurotransmitters responsible for enhancing your overall feeling of well-being, good will, and zest for life is serotonin—by far the most extensively studied neurotransmitter. It influences practi-cally every aspect of life, helping to shape your mood, energy level, memory, sex drive, and outlook on life. It increases your ability to concentrate on a particular subject or problem for extended periods of time, to care about the problem, and to look at the challenges with hope. Serotonin also provides you with deeper and more rest-ful sleep.

Greater serotonin activity is linked to better mood, reduced appetite, more physical energy, and more resilience to stress. When your serotonin is high, you are apt to be relaxed, brimming with energy and loving life. When serotonin is low, you are apt to be low and going lower still; life looks bleak and feels worse. It is difficult to concentrate or calm down, and sleep is fitful. People with low levels of serotonin are more vulnerable to depression, impulsive acts, alcoholism, overeating, suicide, aggression, and violence.

Peacekeeping serotonin fluctuates widely with your monthly cycle. Estrogen is a precursor to serotonin and boosts its production in the brain. When estrogen levels are high, women have more serotonin activity — a potent antidote to the symptoms of hormonal havoc. Antidepressants such as Prozac work by enhancing serotonin. Estrogen works in the brain like a natural Prozac, keeping serotonin from being reabsorbed by other cells, so its effects last longer. Thereby, as our bodies manufacture less estrogen, serotonin may also be in short supply, producing mood changes, restless sleep, and anxiety. Women have low levels of estrogen in the days before menstruation (a partial explanation of PMS), after giving birth (a partial explanation for postpartum depression), while breast-feeding, and during perimenopause and the years following menopause.

Estrogen and progesterone impact serotonin production dramatically, which is why hormone imbalance results in faulty serotonin response. But even HRT does not totally override a chemical imbalance in the brain.

Supplemental hormones by the bucketful won't balance your hormones if you are chronically exposed to extreme, unresolved stress, poor diet, and no exercise. Are you beginning to grasp why achieving hormone balance is about achieving *life* balance?

In order for our bodies to produce levels of hormones and brain chemicals adequate to support our health and well-being during menopause, we must be optimally healthy going in — emotionally, spiritually, and physically.

The Hormone Balancing Plan coming in part 3 is designed to help you get to that place of vitality and wholeness, nourishing your body and spirit to meet the never-ceasing demands of life. But before we jump to that plan, if you are like many women, you may want first to find immediate answers for some of the symptoms you are experiencing — and the natural solutions to be employed to bring your haywire hormones into harmony.

HORMONES GONE HAYWIRE TO HORMONES IN BALANCE

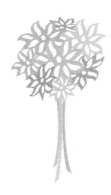

MIDLIFE MALADIES
AND NATURAL SOLUTIONS

In part 1 we contrasted design and disease and considered the differences between menopause and diabetes. There are also similarities. With diabetes, some people have the ability to manage a mild case with lifestyle changes alone—healthy eating, exercise, and good self-care. Others require medication and even insulin to survive. Likewise, in menopause, some women can manage their symptoms with lifestyle changes. Others cannot—and not because they are failures or basket cases, but because the immediate hormonal imbalance is just too intense. There is no shame in getting your needs properly met. Seeking help is to be applauded.

For some women, a short term use of Hormone Replacement Therapy (HRT) may be necessary to calm their hormonal storm. It was originally developed to treat these symptoms. Your doctor may recommend that you go on HRT, at least temporarily, because there's good evidence that these drugs, which maintain your estrogen supply, can help reduce extreme perimenopausal and menopausal symptoms, may protect against osteoporosis, and, for some women, may help avert depression. HRT can be lifesaving—or certainly feel that way.

Take Sheila, for example. She says you would have to wrestle her to the ground to get her hormone prescription away from her; she wants it right next to her in her coffin when she is buried. Her husband heartily agrees; HRT seemed to be the only vehicle that could bring Sheila's hormonal hurricane—and her moods—into balance. She felt she had tried it all: nutrition, exercise, supplemental vitamins and herbs, even antidepressants; but nothing could right the wrong within her body except adequately supplementing with estrogen and progesterone.

Elsie feels the same way, and she should. She had a total hysterectomy at age fifty-two and went into overnight artificial menopause; it hit her with the force of a level-five tornado. Estrogen replacement was an absolute necessity for her; now at eighty-three, she wouldn't consider trying life without it. She says it's a quality of life issue for her. And truly, if I could be promised even a hint of Elsie's vitality and spunk at eighty-three with no risks, I just may sign up for HRT in a heartbeat!

But not every woman can or should take HRT. And some simply don't want to. I'll discuss this more thoroughly in the next chapter. Many women fear the side effects of HRT; others fear the increased risk of cancer and heart disease. Some women simply believe that a more natural approach, using dietary and lifestyle changes, makes better sense for them.

This was the case for Valerie from chapter 1, who balked at taking the pill to stabilize her perimenopausal hormone levels. Like many women her age, she made a decision early on that HRT was not for her—not for menopause, and certainly not now, when that might be years away. She first went on the pill at sixteen; she went off it at twenty-six after two irregular pap smears and after fighting nausea and fluid retention for the whole ten years. Adding to her bad experience, breast cancer had struck her mother and aunt; with those genes she certainly didn't want any increased risk hanging over her. Nor did she want to deal with even more mid-section weight gain than she already had, and that seemed to be a given for all her friends on HRT. So her first line of attack was to look for nutrition solutions and lifestyle enhancements that could calm her hormonal storm.

Valerie, Sheila, eighty-three-year-old Elsie, and countless other clients have all found that healthy eating and exercise can right the wrongs of their personal hormone havoc, either working alone or with supplemental hormones. They have discovered that what they eat—and don't eat—along with their other lifestyle choices has a major impact on how they look and feel during these years marching up to menopause. They also want to invest in the years beyond.

Even though estrogen metabolism is vital to keeping the wiring in harmony, the reality is that hormone treatment alone is not the final answer for any of us. Hot flashes cannot be totally eliminated by HRT as long as your body's blood sugars are allowed to fluctuate wildly. All the hormone replacement in the world—natural or synthetic—won't be enough to control your body's chemical gymnastics if your brain's production of serotonin is being blocked. By learning about the breakthrough research regarding brain function and body chemistry, you will come to understand that through stabilizing your body chemistries, relief is at hand. And it doesn't take a degree in endocrinology or neuroscience to get it. There truly are natural, everyday solutions to your present-day maladies! Just take a look at the following chart—it's help at a glance. Don't let some of the unfamiliar terms concern you; the chapters that follow will explain them in detail.

Notice the common ground with the remedies on the next page, regardless of the symptom, are *lots of water, eat well and often, exercise, sunshine, whole grains and fiber, smart fats, phytoestrogens*—simple strategies that yield tremendous payoff. It's one of the many miracles of our creation; we were designed to thrive with proper nourishment, movement, fresh air, sunlight, and rest. They are God-given instruments of wellness and of healing.

I'll go into much more detail about how to implement each of these power points in Part 3 of this book, "Your Twelve-Week Plan for Hormonal Balance." But first, we will look at pros and cons of Hormone Replacement Therapy. Then we will examine the "what and why" of each of these symptoms and give a quick overview of the solutions—the ways you can restore your well-being by bringing your hormones and brain chemistries into balance. My goal is to equip you with the tools to be your very best in midlife—overcoming pesky symptoms safely and naturally.

Midlife Maladies and Natural Solutions

Symptom	Solutions
achy joints	plenty of water, increased omega–3s and other essential fatty acids; phytoestrogens
cravings	small, frequent meals and snacks of whole carbohydrates and lean proteins—and lots of water
constipation	high fiber foods, 30–35 grams of fiber daily—and lots of water
depression	eat well, eat often; increased omega–3s, B vitamins, magnesium; sunlight
dry skin and hair	frequent protein; essential fatty acids; fruits and vegetables—and lots of water
fatigue	eat well, eat often; adequate protein and iron; exercise; sunshine—and lots of water
fluid retention	plenty of water; balanced eating, adequate protein, B vitamins; proper sodium intake
fuzzy thinking, memory loss	eat well, eat often; omega–3s, B vitamins, magnesium; increased fruits and vegetables—and lots of water
headaches	lowered fat intake; adequate riboflavin, calcium and magnesium; eat well, eat often—and lots of water
hot flashes, night sweats	phytoestrogens; vitamin E; eat well, eat often—and lots of water
indigestion, heartburn	small frequent meals of low-fat foods; water after food, not on empty stomach; avoid orange juice and tomato sauce
irritability, mood swings	small, frequent, balanced meals; adequate B vitamins; omega–3s; exercise in sunlight
low libido	phytoestrogens; eat well, eat often—and lots of water; exercise in sunlight
sleep disturbances	eat well, eat often; exercise in sunlight; drink water through day; avoid alcohol within 4 hours of bedtime, caffeine within 8; have whole grain cereal and milk before bed
slow metabolism	eat well, eat often; exercise/strength train—and lots of water
urinary tract infections	avoid sugar; eat well, eat often; drink lots of water; cranberry juice
vaginal dryness	drink water, drink water, drink water; adequate protein; soy and vitamin E

Hormone Replacement Therapy: The Answers Are In

Few things are more upsetting than having to revise your beliefs, especially when your own physician may have encouraged those beliefs and an array of experts cite scientific evidence to back them up.

In July 2002, the Women's Health Initiative, the best study so far of hormone replacement therapy (HRT) in healthy women, showed that the treatment actually increases the risks of heart disease and breast cancer, outweighing any protection against fractures and colon cancer. True, the study showed that if taken for less than four or five years, hormone therapy is a reasonably safe way to deal with menopausal symptoms. But this is a far more modest benefit, overall, than most women had been led to expect.

Now women are asking, "What should I do?" and "Have I done myself damage in taking this stuff?" The answer to the first question is complicated; thankfully, the answer to the second is probably no.

HOW WE GOT HERE

About two out of five postmenopausal American women are on hormones, or were until that summer—a trend that began its upward trajectory some thirty years ago. Hormone therapy comes in two types: estrogen alone (ERT) or the combination of estrogen and progestin, known as HRT. The idea that taking estrogen after menopause helps protect women against osteoporosis has been well established. And there's logic to the idea that it should also protect against cardiovascular disease. Numerous studies have found benefits. Moroever, hormone therapy can counteract unpleasant (and occasionally unbearable) menopausal symptoms, such as hot flashes, vaginal dryness, night sweats, and mood swings.

There are many other reasons why hormone therapy has been so popular — optimism (false as it may be) being only one of them. There were claims (totally unfounded) that it would keep a woman "forever feminine" and "forever young." The companies that made the hormones helped promote such notions, and the media quickly joined the parade. Understandably, women want to stay healthy into old age, especially now that it's reasonable to expect to live thirty or more years past menopause. Doctors were (and are) eager for medications that will help.

Until recently many doctors simply told women: "Take this. You'll look better. You'll feel better." Women did; there was no questioning, especially with the implication that if we didn't take HRT, we were in for hip fractures, saggy and wrinkled skin, dry hair, vaginal dryness — and no sex drive. Who wants that?

The bottom line is that we all just want to feel great, look great, and live great — for life! But we don't want to trade one curse for another, especially when that curse may be fatal.

What Do Women Want?

Sigmund Freud lamented that he had spent a lifetime of practice trying to discover what women really want, all to no avail. Funny, it seems pretty clear when it comes to hormonal harmony! About 75 percent of women have perimenopausal symptoms that are uncomfortable enough to cause them to seek relief, whether through supplemental hormones, dietary changes, exercise, or alternative therapy. When women were asked what they wanted most from these remedies, they listed these as their top ten desires:

1. improved energy
2. weight control
3. convenience and ease
4. maintenance of youthful skin tone
5. confidence in ability to fulfill daily obligations
6. control of hot flashes
7. alleviation of mood swings
8. easy and enjoyable sex
9. natural ingredients
10. maintenance or enhancement of sex drive

All along, however, there were questions about HRT. Does it increase the risk of breast cancer? How about ovarian cancer? Does it protect against heart disease and Alzheimer's? One thing was always missing: a large-scale, well-designed clinical trial that tested the safety and effectiveness of hormone therapy as a way to prevent disease in healthy women. No matter how carefully conducted, all the studies had been observational. That is, they followed groups of women taking hormones and recorded outcomes—a valuable kind of research, but never definitive. These observational studies found that women taking HRT tended to have lower rates of heart disease, stroke, colon cancer, and osteoporosis. It now appears, at least in terms of cardiovascular disease, that these women may simply have been more well to begin with and more likely to see a doctor and lead healthier lives. This, rather than HRT, is what benefited their hearts.

Good and Bad Estrogens

Estrogen is not one hormone but several grouped together, including estradiol, estrone, and estriol. All three estrogens have the same beneficial effects on our skin and vagina and protect the heart and bones.

The estrogens vary in strength. Estradiol is eighty times more potent than estriol and estrone is twelve times stronger than estriol. It's the liver's job to convert estradiol (the more carcinogenic estrogen) first into estrone (less carcinogenic) and then into estriol (which is noncarcinogenic).

Each estrogen is active at different stages of our reproductive lives. Estradiol is active during our adolescent years, but as menopause approaches production of it declines. Around this time the adrenal glands and estrogen-producing fat cells are producing estrone instead.

Classic HRT is based on the estradiol form of estrogen. Critics maintain that it is unnaturally adding the substance at precisely the time the body is naturally reducing its supply of estradiol.

At last, the National Institutes of Health began the needed clinical trial, called the Women's Health Initiative. In part of this study, women were randomly assigned to take HRT (Prempro, the most popular mix of estrogen and progestin) or a placebo. The trial was to have lasted eight and a half years, but was terminated after a little more than five years to protect the participants from further risk, specifically the rising risk of breast cancer.

WHAT THE WHI STUDY FOUND

The Women's Health Initiative found that long-term use (five or more years) of hormone replacement therapy combining the two hormones, estrogen and progestin, *increased* women's risk of heart disease, stroke, blood clots, and breast cancer. The hormones did indeed lower women's risk of bone fractures and colorectal cancer, but only while on the hormones.

The increased risk is very slight, but very real. To put it in numbers: If 10,000 women were taking HRT for a year and 10,000 women were not taking HRT, in the HRT group eight more women would develop invasive breast cancer, seven more would develop heart disease, eight more would have a stroke, and eight more would develop blood clots. There would also be six fewer colorectal cancers and five fewer hip fractures.

How do these numbers relate to your personal decision? Every woman is unique, and no one should start or stop medication without consulting with her doctor. That said, here are some facts that may help you and your doctor arrive at a decision.

Menopause: Most experts today say the benefits of HRT for those women experiencing extreme symptoms of hot flashes, insomnia, mood swings, and vaginal dryness outweigh the risk if hormones are taken for a brief period of time. But if you have been on HRT for several years, or if you started HRT before ever experiencing bothersome symptoms, consider talking with your doctor about tapering off the hormones. You may be surprised. The symptoms you dread may not affect you at all, especially if you exchange a healthier lifestyle for the HRT.

Heart disease: Women taking standard HRT to prevent heart disease should talk with their doctors about gradually discontinuing the medication. The latest research clearly indicates that HRT does not prevent heart disease; rather, it increases a woman's risk.

The reality is that lifestyle change — not HRT — is the best choice for lowering cholesterol and blood pressure, thereby reducing, not increasing, the risk of heart disease for many women.

Osteoporosis: Research shows that HRT does lower a woman's risk of bone fractures. If you are taking HRT to prevent osteoporosis, discuss your family history and treatment options carefully with

Summary of Findings

Here is a summary of major findings by a government health study on women's hormone therapy over the past two years:

July 2002: Government-backed Women's Health Initiative study of 16,608 women is halted because researchers discover significant health risks for women taking estrogen-progestin pills. Risk of heart disease is 29 percent higher than expected. Breast cancer risk increases by 26 percent. Within a year, prescriptions for hormone therapy dropped from ninety million to fifty-seven million.

July 2002: A study of 44,000 women taking estrogen only found that these women had a 60 percent higher risk of ovarian cancer than women who had never used estrogen. Those on the hormone therapy for twenty years or more were three times as likely to develop ovarian cancer as women who did not take it at all. Women who took estrogen for ten to nineteen years had an 80 percent higher risk than nonusers.

March 2003: Hormone replacement therapy fails to improve older women's memory, sleeping, or mental outlook, as many had assumed.

May 2003: Those who took estrogen-progestin an average of more than four years face double the risk of Alzheimer's or other forms of dementia.

June 2003: Breast cancer linked to estrogen-progestin pills may be fast-growing and hard to detect.

August 2003: The risk of heart attacks during the first year on the pills is nearly double the expected rate. Risk is also higher than expected for those with elevated levels of bad cholesterol.

February 2004: Hormone supplements linked to asthma. A study found that women who use hormones during menopause run double the risk of developing the respiratory ailment.

March 2004: Government-backed Women's Health Initiative study of estrogen-only use with 11,000 women is halted because researchers discover that estrogen alone increased the risk of stroke as much as estrogen-progestin does. For every 10,000 women, those taking hormones suffer eight more strokes per year than nonhormone users. There was no increased risk of breast cancer or overall heart disease detected from estrogen-only use.

March 2004: Neither type of hormone therapy seems good for women's brains. Preliminary data from a related study of women sixty-five and older suggest those taking estrogen alone were more likely to suffer some degree of dementia than those taking a placebo.

So many of the presumptions about hormones, as they come to trial, simply do not show evidence of benefit.

your doctor. Questions to consider include: What other treatments can preserve bone health as well as HRT without the risk? What lifestyle changes (such as diet and weight-bearing exercise) can preserve your bone health? Read more about building and keeping strong bones in chapter 13.

Urinary incontinence: Doctors had long assumed that hormone replacement would help older women who suffered from urinary incontinence. But now two trials have shown no improvement, and there may even be a worsening.

Memory loss/dementia/Alzheimer's: The hope that HRT would prevent memory loss and retard the progression of Alzheimer's disease is dimming as well, with clinical trials having shown no benefit in early Alzheimer's disease, and others showing an increase in memory loss and dementia in those on HRT.

Depression: Similarly, there is no evidence that supplemental hormones can treat major depression in postmenopausal women. But hormones may improve "mood and well-being" in women who are suffering from hot flashes and night sweats that disturb their sleep.

IS ANY OTHER HORMONE SAFER?

Unfortunately, no one knows for sure. About twenty million American women still take some form of estrogen therapy—in pills, patches, or creams—but few of these treatments have been carefully studied for long-term risks.

The standard HRT that increased risks in the Women's Health Initiative is conjugated equine estrogen (made from mare urine) at 0.625 milligrams a day, combined with a synthetic progestin called medroxyprogesterone acetate at 2.5 milligrams a day. (Women who have their uteruses must take a progesterone with estrogen because estrogen alone increases the risk of uterine cancer.) This combination is sold under many brand names: Prempro, Premphase, Femhrt, Activella, and Ortho-Prefest.

Some HRT prescription products have fewer side effects than others, particularly estrogens made from micronized estradiol, estrone, or estriol, and "natural" progesterone. These products are not considered "natural" because of their source (they are not found in nature in this form), but because of their chemical composition, which is similar to what the body produces on its own. These "natural" estrogens (estradiol, estrone, and estriol) are available in compounded formulations called triple natural estrogen (TriEst) or dual natural estrogen (BeEst). Natural progesterone is also available in a compounded formulation. Some drug companies also make so-called natural estrogen products, such as Estrace, a pill, and Estraderm, a skin patch; these products contain only estradiol.

Natural estrogens and progesterones have long been touted by alternative health practitioners to be safer and easier to tolerate than traditional high-dose hormones made by drug companies, such as Premarin or Prempro. More doctors are also recommending natural hormones as they are becoming increasingly open to their patients' concerns and suggestions about nutrition and other natural menopause remedies. You should know that today there is nothing one-size-fits-all about hormonal treatment. But you

Summary of Other Options

Here's a summary of what's known—and not known—about other options:

Low-dose HRT: Some doctors believe that lower doses of HRT can offer the benefits without the risks. Studies do indicate that lower doses of estrogen and progestin (about half the dose as in Prempro) can relieve hot flashes and vaginal dryness. Theoretically, lower doses may pose less risk to breast tissue and heart health, but studies have not yet been done.

Estrogen alone: Women who have had their uteruses removed through hysterectomy can take conjugated equine estrogen supplements without progestin. We've known for years that taking estrogen alone can increase the risk of uterine cancer, which is why women who have their uteruses also take progestin. Yet, a new release from the Women's Health Initiative indicates that women who take estrogen also increase their risk of ovarian cancer. Researchers observed that the risk rose the longer the women were on estrogen.

Bio-identical estrogen patches, creams, or vaginal rings: These forms of estrogen are closer to the estrogen naturally produced by a woman's body and are effective against hot flashes and vaginal dryness. Also, they help build bone. They're sold under the brand names Estraderm, Climara, Vivelle, and Alora. Theoretically, estrogen delivered through the skin, thus bypassing the liver and digestive system, may pose less risk to breast tissue and cardiovascular health. However, studies have not yet been done to definitively answer the question.

should also know that, in light of recent findings, other doctors and researchers do not consider natural hormones a safe alternative.

The bottom line: No one really knows. We know less about these natural products than we do about the ones that have been studied. There are no credible controlled studies existing on the effects or safety of natural hormone creams. They might be better, they might be worse.

Research results on some natural preparations, such as natural progesterone cream, has shown questionable effectiveness. It increases saliva levels of progesterone but not blood levels, and it can still increase risk of breast cancer. This makes it a highly controversial treatment. *The motto here is that just because it's natural does not mean it is always better or safer.*

However, prescription hormones come in a variety of formulations, and if you need something fine-tuned for you, your doctor or other licensed medical practitioner can customize a prescription that is filled through a compounding pharmacy. Such pharmacists will work with your doctor to create a product specifically designed for your body chemistry.

WEIGHING THE HRT PROS AND CONS

While estrogen may offer some women a two-for-one benefit—reducing physical and emotional symptoms—it is no longer considered the treatment of choice for every menopausal woman suffering from depression, vaginal dryness, or hot flashes. Taking estrogen, usually combined with progesterone, for a few months or a year or two during the most dramatic time of menopause can surely ease the normal symptoms. But there are trade-offs. Beyond the threat of increased disease risk, many women also experience side effects, including breakthrough bleeding or spotting, water retention, breast tenderness, and cramps. For this reason, as many as six out of ten women who start HRT quit within the first year, according to the North American Menopause Society. Then, a fourth of those who stop go back on to get relief from unstoppable hot flashes and mood swings.

Each of us must carefully weigh the benefits and risks of HRT for our specific symptoms. Consulting our primary care physician, gynecologist, and/or a mental health professional is vital to making the best decision. Questioning their recommendations and comparing and contrasting them is important as well. Such factors as the specific symptoms, the medical and emotional history, and the family's medical history are very important.

If a woman has a strong family history of osteoporosis, HRT could be prescribed, but there are other treatments that may be safer and more effective. By contrast, if there is a strong family history of breast cancer or heart disease, HRT is ill advised. If you do not feel at peace with the course of therapy being prescribed, seek out a second opinion.

What is beyond doubt is that all the answers about hormones won't be here tomorrow, and women have to make decisions today. The emerging consensus holds that if a woman is suffering unbearable hot flashes and mood swings, she may want to consider *short-term* use of HRT and in the smallest dose needed to control the symptoms.

Examine your quality of life and the impact that perimenopausal symptoms such as hot flashes, vaginal dryness, and mood swings may be having on you. Evaluate personal risk factors for heart disease and osteoporosis. Although simple lifestyle changes can be powerful medicine, if you have not had success controlling extreme symptoms through lifestyle changes and if you are at low risk for some

HRT Question Checklist

If HRT is offered as an option to you, here are some issues to discuss with your health care provider before you agree to try it.

☐ Has a thorough evaluation of my hormone levels been done?

☐ Are there lifestyle changes I can make as a first course of treatment?

☐ Which medication is recommended, and which of my symptoms will it alleviate? Has my doctor prescribed this medication to many women my age, with symptoms like mine, and what have been the results?

☐ Based on my family health history and my own risk factors, is this a safe course of therapy?

☐ How long will I need to take hormone replacement, and how soon should I expect relief?

☐ Are there any side effects I can expect? If so, what can I do to minimize them, and how long might they last?

☐ What enhancements can I make in my lifestyle to complement the action of this medication?

☐ If this trial does not relieve my symptoms, what is the next plan of action?

of the possible side effects of HRT (such as breast cancer and heart disease), then using temporary HRT in a small dose may be a good choice for you. If you find you need supplemental hormones in order to reestablish physical and emotional balance, don't see it as a personal failure. You may want to consider a short term "spritz" of hormone therapy (Hormone Spritz Therapy) — just enough to supply you with the tools you need for comfort and well-being, and no more.

Hot flashes have been shown to diminish after three to six months even without treatment, though they may not go away entirely for four to five years. So if you use supplemental hormones, try to taper off the drugs and stop every year or two to see if you can get by without them.

No matter what your personal decision for or against HRT, there are certain things all of us should be doing at midlife to stay healthy and active for as long as we can. They include:

1. Taking stock of yourself and asking, "What do I need to do to make these the best — the healthiest — years of my life?" Don't plan to be old — even in your seventies!

2. Thinking of menopause symptoms as your body's signal to reflect on what you're going to do with the second half of your life and planning action steps to take this very day.

3. Finding a doctor who's on your wavelength and making sure your doctor is telling you both the pros and cons of taking HRT and personalizing it to your particular family and health history.

4. Exploring the many options available, if you do decide to take HRT to relieve your symptoms and give you the long-term health benefits you're looking for. There isn't one product or formulation that's right for everyone. Consider HRT as complementary to your lifestyle medicine — possibly temporary, possibly long-term, only in the dosage needed for your unique situation.

5. Making a healthy lifestyle the very foundation of treating yourself well — in midlife and beyond. Self-care is not selfish; it is the only way you can continue to give. It is the gift to yourself that keeps on giving!

Naturally, all of us want the beneficial effects of estrogen—soft skin, strong bones, a healthy heart, and positive moods—without upping other health risks. Sound impossible? Well, it's not.

Even with your ever-changing estrogen levels, you can reduce your risks for heart disease and osteoporosis by eating a good, low-fat diet (with plenty of fruits and vegetables), getting regular exercise, and using foods (such as soy and flaxseed) that naturally ease your transition to lower estrogen levels. At the same time, pay attention to the messages your body is sending. It is asking for more than a prescription or supplement. Listen to and acknowledge those inner needs that are creating such outward symptoms.

THE BOTTOM LINE

You cannot ignore the hormone issue. You must address your changing body to provide and protect yourself. The stabilizing tools of the Hormone Balancing Plan will equip you to do just that.

If you are a healthy postmenopausal woman who is taking HRT solely to prevent chronic disease, it makes sense to stop. But talk with your doctor.

If you choose to stay on HRT, ask your doctor to reevaluate you once a year to look at risk versus benefits. Remember, hormones are strong drugs. Staying on hormones longer than five years is no longer advisable.

If you choose to stop HRT, taper off the hormones in a gradual weaning process Quitting is especially difficult for women who have been taking hormones for ten years or more. Some women suffer symptoms of withdrawal if they stop abruptly. In fact, quitting cold turkey can bring on "rebound" effects from the quick withdrawal of the hormones, which can include tremendous hot flashes, excessive bleeding, and sleep difficulties—just about worsening every menopausal symptom. Sudden drops in the hormone levels put the body into an "overnight menopause." But if you ease off slowly, you'll probably experience significantly fewer side effects. If you still have withdrawal symptoms despite careful tapering, talk to your doctor about medications to control hot flashes or other problems.

Here is a note I received from Joanie:

Almost two years ago, I went off of HRT after being on it for six years. It was indeed difficult, but not as much as for many of my friends who went off cold-turkey. The tapering off regimen together with the hormone balancing plan seemed to help me ward off the hot flashes, sleep well, and feel well in general—actually better than when I was on the hormones.

If you are among the eight million women still on hormone therapy and would like to stop, there's good news. A Kaiser Foundation study showed that only one in four women in the group that came off hormone therapy went back on to ease debilitating withdrawal symptoms such as hot flashes. At least 75 percent had no symptoms at all or deemed those they had to be mild to tolerable. Of course, it also means that 75 percent of these women who were on hormones didn't have a very good reason to be on them with respect to their own comfort level.

FDA has made it clear in their labeling, and many physicians and professional organizations, including the American College of Obstetrics and Gynecology and the North American Menopause Society, agree that women should go on the lowest effective dose for the shortest possible time and then reassess.

Similarly, for women who are going back on hormones, the recommendation is to go back on to a lower dose and

If you and your doctor agree (I emphasize again—you *must* consult your doctor) that the inconvenience or possible risks of HRT outweigh the benefits for you, here's the right way to stop:

- *Split them up.* If you take combination HRT with estrogen and progesterone in the same pill, ask your doctor for separate prescriptions for each. That way, you can adjust the level of each hormone individually.
- *Reduce estrogen in halves.* Take half of your usual dose for three weeks, and then cut that dose in half for another three weeks. In another three weeks, take that dose every other day, then stop all together.
- *Continue the progesterone.* If you take combination HRT, keep taking your full dose of progesterone, which can help prevent excessive bleeding. Then stop it a month or two after you stop the estrogen, weaning off the same way.
- *Start eating phytoestrogens.* You'll read more about these hormone balancing powerhouses in later chapters, but adding these foods to your diet will cushion you with plant estrogens already circulating in your system before you are off HRT completely, helping to ward off rebound effects.

then try again to slowly come off to reassess the need for the hormones.

Here's a note from Suzie, an example of a lady who is very grateful for hormone therapy and sees it as "well worth the risks" for the quality of life it is providing her:

> I'm 45 years old and work for a chiropractic physician and have for 6 years now. At age 40, I lost weight down to 130 lbs for my 5'5" frame; I exercise daily but not extremely. I have diabetes, but it's controlled by diet and exercise.
>
> My menstrual cycles started to get funky, and blood work showed I was clearly in perimenopause. I slowly fell off the good eating wagon, and left behind *all* the things I should for a natural trip through this phase of my life.
>
> My body was changing. I had everything on the list—from a dried-up body and hot flashes to mood swings and fatigue. I had to go down to only working 2 days a week. I cried all the way home every night. My doctor suggested Wellbutrin (an anti-depressant), and I tried it for 2–3 months, with no noticeable effects. Then, another antidepressant with a different name. Nothing. Next, natural hormone cream: TriEst and progest. My breasts got so sore I couldn't bear it. Blink. There went another try.
>
> My poor family had a really wacko mom and wife who was not functioning normal at all. I would refer to it as "The Blue Funk"—like the worst PMS ever lasting forever.
>
> One and a half years ago, my OB-GYN wanted to try me on a low dose birth control pill, but I refused, saying I wanted to do the natural thing, as I am so known for. Well, I finally went to the OB-GYN again this spring, and after listening to me ever so kindly, he suggested I try Premphase, the very thing I despised. But I was ready to check out of this world, so I became very open.
>
> I read on the Internet and every other place I could about all the risks, and I certainly don't like knowing that I am taking something with so many. But I am alive and can plan my daughter's wedding in August and enjoy life once again. I felt better the day I started taking it and I am blown away at the difference in my life it had made. I felt as if I was getting Alzheimer's like my mom had.
>
> Please understand that I am a well read and educated lady. I ask that that you understand that some people like myself just may need HRT in order to have a life worth living, even with the risks.

My encouragement to Suzie was to use the HRT and yes, celebrate the life it is providing her. But I also suggested she understand she needs it for the now, possibly not forever. After six months (and getting through her daughter's wedding!), it would be advisable to start tapering down on the hormones, while at the same time "up the ante" on her commitment to the Hormone Balancing Plan (in light of her diabetes, especially in the area of stabilizing her blood chemistries). Most importantly, I want Suzie to not be gripped by fear or guilt for using HRT.

Here's another note — from Rebecca, age forty-nine:

> My doctor wasn't surprised when I chose to forego HRT, nor was she argumentative when I told her that I saw this as a way of honoring my body and the natural changes going on within me. At the same time, I wanted to provide my body with support and help it adjust, so my symptoms wouldn't be severe or interfere with my living life well.

Rebecca chose to provide that support through strategic nutrition, focused exercise, and plant-based hormones (phytoestrogens). There are sensible and safe solutions, just like those Rebecca is using, to achieving hormone balance. A life strategy for eating and fitness can become a lifelong blueprint for healthy living.

Hot Flashes, Night Sweats, and Heart Palpitations

Second only to weight gain, hot flashes are the most frequent symptom associated with menopause. Some studies show that up to 85 percent of women experience hot flashes at some time during their perimenopausal years. They can be mild or they can be so severe that they interrupt sleep and productivity, leading to mood swings and depression.

If you've had a flash, you know exactly what I'm describing. It may just be a passing feeling of warmth in the face or upper body, or it may be a shower of sweat followed by chills. When flashes occur with drenching perspiration during the night, they're called night sweats. Feelings of anxiety and tension may precede the flash, and an increased heart rate, tingling in the hands, dizziness, or nausea may accompany it. Some women experience heart palpitations as well, which can be frightening if unexpected.

IS IT A POWER SURGE?

Although their cause is not totally understood, it seems that flashes (also known as *vasomotor flushing*) are simply the midlife body's way of cooling itself down. Some have theorized that they are a necessary part of the midlife rewiring of the brain or a creative burst of energy. Whatever their purpose, it is generally accepted that abrupt changes in the body's "thermostat" in the brain (the hypothalamus) can cause it to mistakenly sense that you are too warm, so blood vessels in the skin of the head and neck open more widely than usual. Blood rushes to the surface of the skin to cool the body, which is why you get the red, flushed look on your face and neck. Sweating helps cool the body too, as the perspiration evaporates—sometimes too much, and you are suddenly chilled to the bone.

It seems that declining estrogen levels and the resulting higher levels of FSH are the primary triggers for the hypothalamus to fire the flash. Hot flashes tend to become more frequent after our periods actually stop—the time when estrogen levels are the lowest and FSH levels are the highest. Interestingly enough, thin women are more apt to be besieged with hot flashes because of the lack of fat stores to help make up the estrogen difference (I'll discuss this further in chapter 16). Extremely overweight women also have more than their share of flashes—a result of *too much* estrogen production from the fat cells. And women who do not sweat easily are also impacted more extremely with hot flashes.

Keep track of your flashes. Knowledge is power. By keeping a written record of them, you may be able to see a pattern develop. You may have flashes around the same time of day, in particular situations, or after a certain food or drink. Predicting flash triggers will help you manage them better.

On the whole, however, predicting when a flash is likely to occur can be difficult. Because the hypothalamus is calling the shots here, albeit incorrectly, anything that triggers a surge of adrenaline is apt to trigger a flash. Eating patterns that fuel wide blood sugar swings—long hours without eating, chemical stimulants from caffeine, sugar, or alcohol, and stressful situations—are all culprits.

For example, night sweats are triggered when the body's blood sugars begin to drop, often at 2:30 to 3:00 A.M. The body reads the chemical gymnastics as life threatening and sends a surge of adrenaline through the body. This surge sends emergency signals to the hypothalamus, waking you with a "start" and causing a misfire of temperature control.

Did You Know?

Exercise helps in just about every case of perimenopausal symptoms, but it is particularly helpful in prompting the body into a more consistent cooling mechanism.

Hot flashes and sweating are not always about menopause. In some cases, they can be indicative of thyroid dysfunction or an infection. When you're having menopausal hot flashes, you may feel tired because you haven't had a good night's sleep, but you shouldn't feel sick. Moreover, a fever should not accompany the sweats.

TURNING DOWN THE THERMOSTAT

Eat often and eat balanced. Keeping blood sugars stable is critical for controlling hot flashes; the chemical gymnastics caused by roller coaster blood sugars are a perfect prescription for triggering a flash. The hormone balancing meal plan—eating several small and balanced meals throughout the day—is your prescription to stop them.

Add in cooling phytoestrogens. There are certain plants (*phyto*) —such as soy, flaxseed, and red clover—that contain estrogen-like substances. It's believed that foods rich in these phytoestrogens are why so few Japanese women (only about 10 percent) report problems with hot flashes at menopause. The traditional Japanese diet contains a great deal of phytoestrogens from soy products, including tofu, tempeh, and miso.

I'll discuss and list these wonder substances in detail in chapter 21. Many studies are underway exploring their stabilizing and preventive role in a myriad of maladies. In the meantime, to relieve hot flashes, try increasing the amount of soy foods and other phytoestrogen-rich foods in your daily intake. Don't go overboard, however; too much of even a good thing may be bad for you. Have no more than three servings a day—and make those whole soy foods, not supplements.

Drink water! Drink water! Drink water! Staying hydrated is vital for managing just about any malady of menopause and is critical for those suffering with hot flashes. In addition to the eight 8-ounce glasses of water you drink each day, drink a glass of cool (not cold) water when you first feel a flash coming on, and you might halt it in its tracks. Keep water by your bed for middle-of-the-night relief.

Also consider carrying a small spray bottle filled with mineral water and use it to mist yourself as if you were a delicate hothouse plant. It soothes hot flashes and, of course, helps hydrate dry skin.

If you smoke, try to stop. Period. The decreased circulation caused by smoking may significantly trigger and add more intensity to the flashes, not to mention all of its other health risks.

Avoid triggers. Many foods and beverages serve as triggers to insulin surges and blood sugar fluctuations, which in turn can trigger a hot flash:

- refined sugars and carbohydrates
- caffeine
- alcohol
- spicy foods
- excess salt in foods

The impact of these stimulants on your whole body—the good, the bad, and the ugly—is discussed in chapter 26. If your Flash Diary reveals that they play a part in your personal heat episodes, you may want to curtail your use of them.

Consider vitamin E supplements. Although there is no clear scientific evidence that vitamin E can provide relief from hot flashes, personal testimonies continue to indicate that it may have some possible effect on the intensity of hot flashes—at least for some women.

Carolyn was sixty-seven when the news about the risks of HRT came out, and she had been taking estrogen for nineteen years, since a total hysterectomy at age forty-eight. She went off the estrogen cold turkey and lived to regret it. She was experiencing fifteen to eighteen hot flashes a day and ten to twelve at night, and nothing seemed to give relief.

She came to me questioning if she'd just have to "live like this." The sleep deprivation was sucking the life out of her. We worked on fine-tuning her balanced, well-timed plan of eating, including a daily dose of phytoestrogens, lots of brightly colored fruits and vegetables, and plenty of water; that alone cut the frequency and intensity in half. We added a supplement of 400 IU vitamin E, and the flashes dropped to none to three per day—and they now seem to stop about the same time she notices one is coming.

Vitamin E is essential to the proper functioning of blood and for the production of sex hormones, which may explain its impact on hot flashes. The best food sources are whole grain cereals and breads, nuts and seeds, green leafy vegetables, dried beans, and olive oil. If you try a supplement, start with 800 IU per day to see if there is an improvement. If so, after three weeks, try just 400 IU, and then cut down to 200 IU to see if there continues to be a protection against the flash. Take the supplement with lunch or dinner. If you have high blood pressure, diabetes, or heart disease, speak with your physician before taking vitamin E. Vitamin E supplements have been shown to increase heart attack risk for those with established heart disease.

Carolyn is now living relatively free of hot flashes and is now down to 200 IU of vitamin E a day.

Go for boron, bioflavonoids, and magnesium. Boron (in broccoli and blueberries), bioflavonoids (in citrus and mangos), and magnesium (in spinach and sunflower seeds) may be helpful to halt the flash because of their help in stabilizing central nervous system stimulation. The "color brightening" step of the Hormone Balancing Plan (chapter 20) will provide you with ample amounts of these nutrients.

Exercise. If you have not found motivation to exercise for any other reason, halting hot flashes may be it. Recent studies show that active women report fewer hot flashes than inactive women. This may be a result of a more trained cooling mechanism that comes through efficient sweating. In addition, routine exercise improves your circulation, which can make the body more tolerant of temperature extremes and better able to cool down quickly. Lastly, exercise strengthens the endocrine system — especially the ovaries and adrenal glands — and seems to increase the amount of estrogen and other hormones circulating in the blood. Refer to chapter 27 to read more about the power of exercise in hormone and blood chemistry stabilization.

Allow yourself to healthfully gain five pounds if you are underweight or a chronic dieter. This means eating well and often, but eating a bit more to nourish the hungry fat cells into becoming bigger and better production sites for estrogen. A healthy weight gain is not a bad thing in perimenopause; it will *greatly* reduce your symptoms. I know this is frightening — gaining weight! — but is one of the more effective strategies for many of my clients.

Pray — possibly the best solution of all. Research has shown prayer and relaxation to relieve hot flashes in about 90 percent of women, with no other therapy. Here is an opportunity to turn a frustration into a positive action. If you experience a hot flash, use it as a reminder to stop and pray right then, thanking God for his marvelous design of the human body. Meditate for a moment on his power and presence—and ask for a calming breeze of peace to cool you.

If hot flashes are debilitating, do not hesitate to talk to your physician about antidepressants or hormone replacement. In one recent study, menopausal breast cancer patients who took about half the standard dose of the antidepressant venlafaxine (Effexor) had a 61 percent reduction in hot flashes. Preliminary results suggest a similar effect with other antidepressants, such as fluoxetine (Prozac) and paroxetine (Paxil).

As you have read, estrogen replacement is amazing when it comes to cooling hot flashes; it has been shown to be about 95 percent effective. For this reason, if hot flashes are drastically interfering with your life and you are not responding to the other natural solutions listed above, using a "spritz" of HRT may be warranted. Indeed, two-thirds of women begin this therapy for hot flash relief. In addition to estrogen replacement, a 2 percent progesterone skin cream also works in about 85 percent of perimenopausal women. Just keep in the mind the possible trade-offs in this choice (see chapter 7).

THE HERBAL CHOICE

Supplements and herbs may have a role in stabilizing hormones, but we must come to understand which therapies from traditional and holistic medicine are effective and which are not. Some menopausal women now take chasteberry to prevent hot flashes, though little research exists to support its effectiveness, and I don't recommend it for this reason. Similarly, avoid dong quai and licorice root. Dong quai can cause excessive blood thinning, while licorice root may precipitate headaches or high blood pressure.

Black cohosh is another story. This herb is used in various products (such as Remifemin or Black Cohosh Power) and remains one of the best-selling herbs for menopausal symptoms. Some women see it as "natural" and prefer it to hormone replacement therapy to deal with hot flashes. In turn, some women claim it also improves their sex drive and eases night sweats and sleep disturbances. Black cohosh can be taken in tablet, capsule, or tincture form. A standardized dosage may be found at health foods stores with a recommended dose of one to two tablets daily (up to 80 mg).

However, as with so many herbal remedies, controlled studies on black cohosh are scant. Some studies have found that it relieves hot flashes, sweating, headaches, and other menopausal symptoms, but few of these studies have been well designed. One three-month study of 976 postmenopausal women found that those who took 40 mg of black cohosh daily reduced symptoms such as hot flashes, mood swings, night sweats, and insomnia compared with those who didn't take the herb. Those findings were presented in 2002 at the annual meeting of The Endocrine Society. Another study published March 28, 2002, in the *Journal of Women's Health and Gender-Based Medicine* found that black cohosh extract, marketed as Remifemin, reduced symptoms in 70 percent of women.

However, overall reviews of published studies on black cohosh have found that research is limited and inconclusive. Some researchers think black cohosh contains plant estrogens and thus has hormonal effects, but the latest reports have found no estrogens or hormonal effects. Regardless, this form of black cohosh (Remifemin) is so widely used in Europe that the German Commission E (that nation's form of the FDA for herbs) has approved its use for hot flash treatment — for up to six months. There have been no studies verifying its safety for longer than this period, and one recent study showed no improvement in symptoms from its use.

There have also been reports that black cohosh may elevate liver enzymes, suggesting it may adversely affect the liver, along with stomach upsets, headaches, dizziness, and weight gain. It's unknown whether black cohosh has any effect, positive or negative, on breast cancer risk. And it is also not clear whether women taking birth control pills or hormone replacement therapy can safely take black cohosh.

For these reasons, and because of my concern about its possible impact on endometrial cancer risk, I do not recommend it as a first course of treatment. Try the other "Turning Down the Thermostat" strategies before black cohosh; try black cohosh before HRT.

Final thoughts: If you try black cohosh, be sure your physician knows. Ask whether it might interact with other medications you are taking. Black cohosh is an interesting herb. Perhaps good studies will one day be done, so that you could be more certain of its benefits and potential side effects. Thus far its traditional uses and benefits have no solid support from scientific research.

HEART PALPITATIONS

Palpitations can feel as if the heart is beating erratically or fast, skipping a beat, or as if there are butterflies in your chest. Usually they occur with hot flashes and night sweats, but they can appear on their own. Like hot flashes, they can range from moderate to severe. They are rarely dangerous, though they can sometimes be frightening. The fluctuating levels of estrogen during perimenopause cause a destabilization of the cardiac rhythm, which can lead to these palpitations.

While palpitations are usually harmless, they may be signs of a serious heart rhythm abnormality or heart disease until proven otherwise. Thus, it should be evaluated for the cause. Even a revved-up thyroid (hyperthyroidism) can increase the effects of adrenaline, a stress hormone in the body, which can cause a rapid heart rhythm or arrhythmia (this can be diagnosed with a TSH test).

If it turns out that palpitations are related to menopausal changes like hot flashes, they can usually be relieved with adequate balancing of hormones, avoiding stimulants, and equalizing blood chemistries. Because they are usually rooted in the stress response system, anything that triggers a stress response—from fear and anxiety to stimulants like MSG, caffeine, sugar, and even dehydration—can trigger palpitations. For this reason, the Hormone Balancing Plan works toward avoiding this kind of stimulation of adrenaline surges and instead focuses on eating and drinking to bring stabilization to the body—and to the heart.

SUMMING IT UP

The very best news of all about perimenopausal hot flashes and palpitations is that they are temporary, not a life sentence. They respond well to lifestyle changes: eating well, exercising, drinking water, relaxation, and prayer—upgrades that will result in much more than just "managing the flash." These steps toward wellness will energize and strengthen you, bringing out the best of yourself for the best in life.

Here's a note from Kathy, who did just that:

> I just turned 51 and am still having periods every month but things are "changing" and personally I really do not want to have to take HRT. I have experienced some hot flashes and vaginal dryness, and just before my periods start, I was seeing that I was far more emotional than I usually was in my younger years during that time of the month. So my symptoms were mild in comparison to what I've heard other women report. Perhaps it is part genetics, but nonetheless following the Hormone Balancing Plan has made such a wonderful difference in the way I feel! I drink lots of water, eat often and well, try to get some daily exercise (walking or an exercise tape for me). I may be 51 by the calendar but I feel 25! I have lots of energy to do all that God has assigned to me (a husband and five great kids!) I am truly thankful!! God bless you all in the work you are doing!

Those Restless Nights

I t's 3:00 A.M., and there you are, laying awake and wondering how in the world you are going to think straight, function, and have energy when your day starts in three short hours.

You went to sleep quickly—dead to the world. But then you awakened with a start, in a puddle of sweat, scared to even look at the clock. When you finally do, it's only 2:00 A.M.—just two and a half hours of sleep logged in. You toss, you turn, and by 3:00 A.M. you are desperate to get back to sleep, knowing what is ahead of you that day. When the alarm finally goes off at 6:00 A.M., you are ready to write your own lyrics to "A Hard Day's Night."

Sleep deprivation is serious at any time of life. But it especially takes its toll during perimenopause, leaving you longing for a good night's sleep as much as a starving person yearns for food. Most often, insomnia at midlife is rooted in night sweats and hot flashes, and as you'll soon learn, these are exaggerated when blood sugars are unstable. Another cause is the lack of serotonin, resulting in an anxiety response that prevents sound sleep.

Anything that triggers a surge of adrenaline will awaken you with a start, and the rush of stress hormones through your body will prevent you from getting back to restful sleep. Thereby, triggers can be the same as those for hot flashes: going long hours through the day without food, eating highly refined carbohydrates and sugar, caffeine, alcohol, lack of exercise, anxiety, and stress.

Actually, it's a wonder that we sleep as well as we do!

The bottom line to a good night's sleep is this: How you live your days is going to have a serious impact on how well you sleep at night. So job one for restful sleep is to focus on stabilizing your body chemistries and hormones during the day. The Hormone Balancing Plan in the next section will get you on the right road, as will these tips to prepare your body for getting the rest you need.

DAYTIME ACTIVITIES THAT PREPARE FOR A GOOD NIGHT

Get outside. The release of hormones in your brain is regulated by the nerve impulses sent by your retinas in response to light. In other words, living by the God-designed natural cycle of light and darkness keeps your serotonin and cortisol at their proper levels. Getting at least thirty minutes of natural light a day helps reset our inner alarm clocks, so we'll want to fall asleep at the right time. Read more about the power of light in chapter 28.

Take a walk. In one study of more than seven hundred people, those women who took daily walks were one-third less likely to have trouble sleeping until their normal wake-up time. Those who walked briskly slashed the risk of any sleep disorder by half. Regular exercise alleviates stress and also raises body temperature, which primes us for better slumber at night. Just be sure not to exercise within an hour of bedtime; it will backfire and charge you up rather than calm you down.

Eat well, eat often. I know this isn't new "news," but it's vital for ensuring sound sleep. Undergird your blood sugars with support by eating small, balanced meals, evenly timed and distributed throughout your day. Keeping your blood sugars up and even through the day prevents surges of stress chemicals and allows for better sleep come nighttime. You'll read all about it in chapter 19.

ABC'S OF GOOD ZZZZS

When it comes to the bedtime hour itself, whether you have trouble falling or *staying* asleep, these tips should help.

Prepare your body for sleep. Breathe easy; deep, slow, mindful breathing can calm you and put your body in the mood for sleep. Relax with a book or restful music. Take a warm bath with Epsom salts, which eases stress and gives a bonus benefit of added magnesium absorption (use one cup Epsom salts for a full bath). Light some candles for natural light—and relax!

Prepare your soul for rest. Pray, recalling the greatest blessings of your day and thanking God for each one! Read an encouraging story or Scripture passage. Reflect on a promise of hope.

Keep the room dark. Darkness stimulates the production of melatonin, a light-sensitive hormone produced by the pineal gland, which is located in the brain (read more about melatonin below). To manipulate this hormone naturally, invest in thick, heavy curtains, or simply don an eye mask.

Keep the room cool. Layer the bedclothes and wear lighter cotton nightclothes.

Curtail spicy foods, caffeine, and alcohol as bedtime elixirs. You may need to avoid caffeine altogether, or at least limit it to before 12:00 noon each day. Try a warm cup of chamomile tea if you are looking for a hot beverage.

Choose your bedtime snack wisely. A bowl of cereal, or banana and milk, will increase levels of serotonin in the brain, making you feel good *and* sleepy, and it will regulate your nighttime blood sugars, keeping you asleep.

Try calcium at bedtime. Calcium is another sleep inducer. If you supplement with calcium, take it before you go to bed rather than in the morning.

Drink your water quota before 5 P.M. This is important if your sleep is being disturbed by middle-of-the-night bathroom trips.

Be aware of sleep-disturbing medications. Be especially careful about allergy medications, decongestants, and certain herbs—even vitamin B6. All can prevent you from going into the deep refreshing sleep that you need.

Let bed be bed. It should not be an office, a bill-paying central, or a home theater. Reclaim bed for sleeping and romance.

Don't force the sleep issue. If you are still awake thirty minutes after going to bed, get up and do something calming, such as reading or praying, until you're groggy

Sleep Elixir

Try this sleep elixir: Warm up a cup of nonfat milk or soy milk and mix it with one teaspoon honey, a dash of vanilla, and a sprinkle of nutmeg, cinnamon, or cardamom. This is also a great drink for putting you *back* to sleep in the middle of the night.

enough to fall asleep. Try to stay awake until your eyes close involuntarily. This works best if you don't keep track of time. Set the clock. If you awaken in the middle of the night and are unable to get back to sleep, avoid obsessively watching the clock. Don't let your mind start racing through to-do lists, guilts, or fears. Focus on a calming prayer or phrase;.count your blessings instead of sheep.

Research shows the better choice is to get to sleep an hour earlier. This practice provides the extra rest without upsetting the rhythm. Stick with it; it can take weeks to make up lost sleep. Also helpful is the afternoon power nap—definitely a snooze you can use! A fifteen- to twenty-minute rest can do wonders for your body. It gives your mental energy a boost, just as it does your physical energy. You

---

Did You Know?

When it comes to catching up on lost sleep, timing is everything. Your body's internal time clock is daily reset by getting up at the same time each day, regardless of when you fall asleep. "Sleeping in," even for an hour or after a bad night's sleep, can disrupt your biological clock and end up making you feel more fatigued.

A Word about Melatonin

Beyond estrogen and serotonin declines, there are other hormones that affect sleep for the perimenopausal woman. Studies show at around age forty, nighttime blood levels of the sleep-regulating hormone melatonin begin to decline.

Although melatonin supplements are commonly used for insomnia or jet lag, the high doses found in most supplements can cause grogginess, nightmares, and impaired functioning when driving and performing other activities. They may actually contribute to hormonal imbalance by triggering secretion of androgens.

In a new study, people with insomnia were given 0.1 mg, 0.3 mg or 3 mg of melatonin. Each dose improved sleep, but the 0.3-mg dose was most successful. The implication is that a bedtime dose of 0.3 mg may be an effective treatment for insomnia. Although it's sold over the counter, ask your doctor about melatonin before taking it; it is a hormone and should not to be taken without awareness of its interplay with other hormones. I do not recommend it to my clients other than for short-term use in traveling across time zones or for temporary bouts of insomnia.

don't even need to sleep; just lying down produces more alertness and less anxiety, confusion, and fatigue in the hours that follow.

Sleeping well and resting well are vital spokes in the wheel of hormone wellness. They are the repair shop of the body and brain, the process that most thoroughly restores our vitality after the strain and exertion of life. More important than just the hours "clocked-in" for sleep, the measure of *restful* sleep is what makes the healthy difference for replenishment. Remember that how well you live your days impacts how well you sleep at night — and, in turn, how well you think and feel the next day.

MENTAL FUZZINESS AND MEMORY LOSS

Many of us feel that we have finally hit our stride in our forties. We're not only the anchors for our families, but we've also advanced in our careers or our own businesses and are making a difference in our communities and churches.

But then, we begin to sense being sidelined by mysterious changes in our memory and brain power. Frequent memory lapses and mental fuzziness not only make our days less productive but rack our self-confidence and leave us wondering who we are.

A common question surfaces: Have I lost my mind, or just my keys? Many women feel a growing sense of forgetfulness and "cotton head" during perimenopause. It's not unusual to have trouble concentrating, to do things like losing your cell phone (only to find it in the freezer), to walk into a room and wonder what you're there for, or to forget why you've called someone (or maybe whom you're talking to!). Hormonal changes can seem to poke holes in your memory and concentration and make you feel as if you are losing your grip. Disturbed sleep and emotional stress can make a bad situation worse.

Once again, the question is: *Is it aging—or my hormones?*

The answer: *a little of both.* Researchers are taking a harder look at the connection between hormone levels and brain function, particularly the role of estrogen in improving memory and concentration. Estrogen has been found to raise acetylcholine production, a chemical that helps us to retrieve information stored in the brain. Thus, as estrogen levels begin to fluctuate and dwindle, brain power can in fact become temporarily inconsistent and scanty.

Estrogen also increases the amount of blood that flows to a woman's brain. It relaxes key arteries, allowing more blood to pass through. When cerebral blood flow is high, people have better memory and are less likely to be depressed. When blood flow to the brain is low, memory, thinking, and moods are compromised.

Stress also comes into play with mental fuzziness because of the estrogen-blocking and memory-blocking action of the stress hormones. Ever flubbed a job interview, suffered a memory lapse during a presentation, or forgotten the boss's husband's name at the company picnic? Stress hormones like cortisol may chemically block the ability to recall some information—just when you need it most. Stress has significant effects on the brain, particularly on memory.

Of course, there's also the stress of wading through the immense "brain glob" that has accumulated in our midlife brains. Although not established in research, brain glob is certainly an issue to take stock of (even jokingly!). Your personal levels can be tested easily: If you can immediately break into the *Gilligan's Island* theme song without missing a word, if you can remember your high school boyfriend's shirt size or your lines from the kindergarten class play, or if you are the reigning Trivial Pursuit champion—you have a whole lot of it. That's the brain glob you have to navigate through when you are trying to simply remember the password for five different security systems and your ATM card!

Some of the memory lapses may be strong hints that we need to pay attention to, as if our bodies are saying, "Slow down! The hard drive is full!" And, some of our "midlife moments" may be simply a matter of being on low-battery—not enough of the high-power food we need for peak performance.

PREMIUM BRAIN FUEL

Food is your primary brain regulator, so be sure to make it the very best it can be! Remember: Neurotransmitters are chemicals produced in the brain to "fire" brain function. The type of neurotransmitters your brain makes and releases plays an all-important role in your mental performance and overall well-being. The levels and potency of these neurotransmitters depend greatly on the quality of food you eat. Your brain cells require a steady supply of energy and certain nutrients as building blocks to make them.

Before you get even more befuddled and overwhelmed at the complexity of it all, let me give you some examples. Your brain cells need tryptophan, an amino acid in foods like whole grains, milk, and turkey, to readily create "happy and calm" serotonin. Similarly, choline, concentrated in eggs and soy, is required to make the neurotransmitter acetylcholine, which is critical for memory, especially in midlife. The brain makes the neurotransmitter dopamine, essential for proper thinking capability and motor coordination, from tyrosine, found in high protein foods such as fish. Other nutrients such as folic acid, vitamin B6, magnesium, and fish oil can help determine the amount, character, and functioning of other brain-enhancing neurotransmitters.

When brain cells don't get enough of the right nutrients at the right time, neurotransmitter systems can go awry with disastrous consequences. Hormonal imbalance follows.

Small wonder that our midlife bodies and brains frequently malfunction, sending us into extreme symptoms of fatigue, sleeplessness, mood swings, depression, memory decline, and hot flashes. Our brains are running on empty because our modern-day diets and lifestyles are so incongruent with our genetic wiring. We feed ourselves processed foods the body can't recognize and can't use while it yearns for premium fueling to energize and protect.

This is why the foundation of the Hormone Balancing Plan is that of eating well and eating often, fueling the brain with a constant supply of high

Power B Foods

Vitamin B6 (needed: 2 mg daily)

Potato	.91 mg
Banana	.73 mg
Whole grain cereal (½ cup)	.50 mg
Lean beef (3 oz.)	.48 mg
Halibut (3 oz.)	.34 mg

Folic Acid (needed: 400 mcg daily)

Chickpeas, cooked (½ cup)	140 mcg
Lima beans, cooked (½ cup)	140 mcg
Spinach, cooked (½ cup)	140 mcg
Orange juice (1 cup)	110 mcg
Strawberries (½ cup)	110 mcg

Vitamin B12 (needed: 6 mcg daily)

Atlantic mackerel (3 oz.)	16 mcg
Beef (3 oz.)	3 mcg
Tuna or salmon (3 oz.)	2 mcg
Milk (8 oz.)	1.5 mcg

quality power meals and snacks to keep your mind sharp, clear, and effective. In addition, there are key ingredients that serve to boost brain power.

Get Bs for the brain. Fuel carriers are also needed to get vital glucose into your brain. These vehicles are the B-complex vitamins, serving as catalysts for the body's important function of utilizing glucose as energy and nervous system fuel. When the brain sputters along without adequate amounts of B vitamins, perimenopausal symptoms intensify, as does depression. Adequate B6, B12, and folic acid are also important to protect the brain from aging free radicals.

Your basic goal is to make foods rich in brain power Bs a part of your daily diet. A daily supplement of 150 mg of B6 can help alleviate perimenopausal symptoms of the "mental type" for many women. If you choose to supplement, limit yourself to less than 300 mg per day; higher levels of supplementation have been linked to serious side effects, such as neuromuscular damage and paralysis. It is generally best to stick to a B complex to cover any needs.

Go fish. Ever hear that fish is "brain food"? That's because, in addition to a boatload of vitamins, minerals, and omega–3 fatty acids, it's an excellent source of the amino acid tyrosine. This amino acid increases the production of dopamine and norepinephrine, which help the body to buffer the effects of stress. Known as catecholamines, these chemicals are considered the "alertness drugs" of the brain. People who get an increase in tyrosine foods perform better at mental tasks and show a significant edge in response time and memory recall. They also experience less anxiety and have more clarity of thought.

Although fish is the single best source of tyrosine and delivers it to you in an almost-no-fat form, all proteins contain this valuable amino acid. However, it's a use-it-or-lose-it nutrient; that is, you have no storage sites for tyrosine or any essential amino acid. This is why eating protein often throughout the day, at least every three to four hours, keeps you bright (in more ways than one!).

Eat your brain chemicals. Choline and inositol (both components of lecithin) are brain chemicals that aid in learning and understanding. When these are low, our brains just don't work as well. Food sources for both include eggs, soy foods, sunflower seeds, wheat germ, oatmeal, brewer's yeast, peanuts, green peas, green leafy vegetables, and lean meat. Inositol is also found in cantaloupe, grapefruit, raisins, and cabbage.

SUMMING IT UP

The bottom line for "clearing brain fog"? Eat well and eat often. A hungry and malnourished brain is simply not a well-performing one! The Hormone Balancing Plan will put it all together for you, giving you the right stuff at the right times for optimum fuel to nourish your body and your mind. The same foods and lifestyle choices that lift the fog from your memory and thinking capabilities also lift the funk that can settle on your moods.

Mood Swings and Body Blues

Mood colors everything we do: what we eat, what we wear, whether we'll make love with our spouse tonight or end up in a disagreement. We all know what it is to be in a great mood: We feel strong and energetic and have an incredible self-image. You love, are lovely, and feel loved; your potential is unlimited, and life is bathed in light.

Bad moods are also easy to identify. You're off, drained of energy, out of control, hating yourself, hating life, hating the people in your life. You have no hope and feel overwhelmed, and everything is dark and dim.

And moods can change in a moment.

Experts in women's health estimate that as many as nine out of ten women suffer from lethargy, mood changes, and other forms of premenstrual discomfort — including fatigue and energy loss. Most women find that a lot of their bad mood days coincide with their menstrual cycle and PMS. Symptoms can be extreme and last a few days or even weeks, and they can occur mid-cycle, right before the onset of their cycle, or both.

These symptoms become exaggerated in perimenopause. Of course, with inconsistent and erratic periods, this is a bit more difficult to ascertain. Again, *is it me or my hormones?*

The answer, more than likely, is *both*.

Although your moods may seem to have no rhyme or rhythm, the ups and downs are often the result of your natural body patterns. The funk you are attributing to hormone fluctuations may be more a result of your daily low points — a drop in energy and heightened tension typical of mid-afternoon and late evening. Bad moods can also be rooted in brain chemical changes from lifestyle and food choices throughout your day. Becoming an observer of your moods will help to track them through the course of your day (and month!) and will show you what impacts them. Generally, bad mood times are very common *and* very preventable.

BEYOND THE BLUES

"I'm really, really depressed, and I know it must be menopause" is a complaint that I hear several times a week from my clients. Truly, perimenopausal women, as a whole, *are* more vulnerable to physical and emotional problems. But unlike a few days of PMS funk, the perimenopausal blues can take bad moods a step further, where they almost take on a life of their own.

The most obvious culprits for dark moods are untreated hot flashes and night sweats. They can leave you feeling irritable and sleep deprived, which may ultimately result in mild depression and loss of your overall sense of well-being. Don't overlook midlife stresses either. Caring for aging parents, raising teenagers, making career changes, or having financial problems often hit at this time and can affect anyone's ability to cope.

When symptoms go beyond normal feelings of sadness and bring on significant changes in weight, social withdrawal, disinterest in life, chronic insomnia, inability to concentrate, and anxiety, they should never be dismissed as "it's just menopause." You could be experiencing a clinical depression.

Depression can result from the abrupt fluctuations—surges and ebbs—of estrogen and progesterone levels in the bloodstream of perimenopausal women. You can have high levels of progesterone and low levels of estrogen one day, and the next day significantly higher levels of estrogen and lower levels of progesterone. As you've already read, these hormone fluctuations cause imbalances in the brain chemical serotonin. This in turn impacts how you feel—emotionally and physically.

Keep in mind that this doesn't mean that depression is inevitable at menopause. But if it does occur, it should be taken seriously and investigated—not brushed off with a "you'll get over it." Depression can also be a symptom of many other disorders, such as low thyroid function.

Women with a history of depression seem to be more vulnerable to another bout of depression at menopause. Thus, it's especially important for a physician to recognize the signs so that treatment isn't delayed. Antidepressant medication and psychotherapy continue to be the treatments of choice, but recent studies show that short-term use of estrogen replacement therapy can reduce symptoms of mild-to-moderate depression in some perimenopausal women without antidepressants. Research has also shown that lifestyle enhancements, such as omega–3 oils and other essential fatty acids, and adequate sunlight can greatly contribute to lifting depression. The Hormone Balancing Plan will equip you to make healthy choices that will make a world of difference in how you feel.

If life and emotions just seem too much to handle, talk with a professional counselor. Shop for the best fit, especially one who values and shares your commitment to spiritual truth.

MOOD FOOD

Omega–3 fatty acids have been shown to regulate periods and to prevent cramps and migraines. A recent study suggests that omega–3 fatty acids found in fish oil may act as a mood stabilizer, providing some short-term relief for sufferers of clinical depression, particularly of the bipolar type. This research was built on a previous finding that people with bipolar disorder, clinical depression, or postpartum mood disorders appear to have lower levels of omega–3 fatty acids in their red blood cells.

Researchers suspect that this fatty acid may inhibit overactive brain-cell signaling. People in countries such as Japan, who eat more foods rich in omega–3 fatty acids (fish like salmon, tuna, sardines, and bluefish as well as flaxseed, walnuts, and dark green leafy vegetables), have a lower incidence of depression. You'll read more about omega–3s in chapter 23.

Chronic emotional and mental stress often results in a magnesium deficiency because the stress hormones cortisol and adrenaline release magnesium from the cells and it is lost. In turn, a low magnesium level can contribute to moodiness and fuzzy thinking.

A well-balanced diet including green leafy vegetables, soy products, nuts, and lots of whole grains is apt to fill your magnesium need. If you supplement, I recommend 350 mg of magnesium per day to lessen the intensity of symptoms. Magnesium gluconate and magnesium aspartate are the most absorbable forms of this mineral.

Beyond eating fish and getting adequate magnesium, there are many other life patterns that can lift and stabilize your moods—even when hormone-related. Remember, it's all about serotonin, so mood-elevating actions are all boosting its production and circulation in the brain, and defending against the impact of cortisol. This means defusing the ever-present stress in our lives. Here are some strategies to do so.

Schedule regular play periods into your appointment book. Whether it's piecing together a puzzle, playing racquetball, or sledding with your kids, play distracts us from our worries and provides a temporary refuge from stress. Golf only counts if it's fun for you rather than just one more competitive stress!

Put mood-stabilizing photos in your "stress zones." In your work area, place beautifully framed pictures of the people you love (or your pet!) to remind you of what's important. Clip to your visor a photo from your last beach vacation to calm you when you're stuck in traffic and lift you up when you are down.

Get a massage. Deep-pressure massage stimulates the nerves that cause our levels of the stress hormones cortisol and epinephrine to go down while the levels of mood-regulating serotonin and dopamine rise. This was true in studies of breast cancer patients, conducted at the Touch Research Institute at the University of Miami School of Medicine, and of women with fibromyalgia and chronic fatigue syndrome. Both groups reported reduced anxiety and depression and improved mood and quality of life.

When a professional massage doesn't fit my budget, I convince my husband that the very best thing he can do for me at the moment is to rub my feet—a loving action that truly can change the direction of my day. Of course, he reminds me that research has also shown that folks who *give* a massage reduce their own levels of stress hormones!

Lift up your eyes. Many of my clients find their best "lift" out of a funk comes through prayer or reading inspirational verses or

Scripture. When meditating on God's peace and blessings, bad moods are banished. Try silently repeating a soothing word or prayer, such as "Peace, be still," while taking slow, deep breaths through your nose, breathing out from your mouth. Consider the excellent advice of the apostle Paul in his letter to the Philippians: "Finally, brothers, whatever is true, whatever is noble, whatever is right, whatever is pure, whatever is lovely, whatever is admirable — if anything is excellent or praiseworthy — think about such things" (Philippians 4:8).

Stay on the sunny side of life. Get out and get some sunshine! One clinically proven, scientifically sound program developed at the University of Washington is called the LEVITY program. A study, reported in 2001 in the journal *Women and Health*, demonstrated that just creating a more natural lighting environment and going outdoors for a brisk twenty-minute walk five or more times a week resulted in women feeling more energetic, having a more positive sense of well-being, and being much less depressed.

Why does the program work? Getting more bright light and engaging in moderate-intensity outdoor exercise reverses many of the physical changes brought about by low or fluctuating hormones and living a light-deprived existence. These activities boost serotonin activity in your brain, increase your cerebral blood flow, and reduce your stress hormones — all adding up to a brighter mood! Sunlight is so important that I have dedicated chapter 28 to it.

Laugh, exercise, make love. The more we do so, the more endorphins our brains release, which results in more serotonin. These "neuro-hormones" — chemicals released in the brain during exercise, deep belly-laughing (and, yes, after lovemaking) — are natural painkillers and also help to alleviate anxiety.

In one study conducted at the Loma Linda University's Center for Neuroimmunology in California, a group who watched a humorous video was found to have 30 percent less of the stress hormone cortisol in their blood and significantly lower levels of epinephrine during and after the tape, compared with a group that sat quietly.

Lighten up your exercise time even more with a cassette or CD of your favorite comedian or a humorous book on tape. Watch out for funny newspaper headlines or ads; watch movies that make you laugh.

And, make time for romance.

Lackluster Libido: Hormones, Vaginal Dryness, UTIs . . . and Your Love Life

When midlife sexual desire sinks, even in the midst of a relationship's romantic sea, the first thing that is to be questioned is your premenopausal status.

The dropping levels of estrogen and the resulting thinning of vaginal tissue, as well as fatigue or adrenal exhaustion, can all be factors in lowered libido. For reasons that are not clear, some women experience a drop in their testosterone levels during perimenopause—another libido buster.

Testosterone is the hormone that fuels sexual desire and enhances pleasure—in women as well as men. As is true for estrogen and progesterone, testosterone levels also vary across the menstrual cycle. Testosterone is low during the first part of the cycle, peaks at ovulation, and then declines during the final two weeks. When a woman has relatively high levels, she is more likely to think about intimacy, respond to a partner's advances, and initiate sex—which is why we were designed for our testosterone to "turn on" at ovulation.

Beyond a drop in libido, there is growing evidence that some of the other perimenopausal symptoms—especially fatigue and anxiety—may be due to a woman's variable supply of testosterone. It often merits a test of your levels. A variety of treatments, including supplements, exercise, eating well, and a focus on soy isoflavones, can make the healthy difference.

VAGINAL DRYNESS

Another blanket on libido is vaginal dryness. In their forties, some women will notice that their vaginas take longer to become lubricated during sexual arousal and may become irritated by the same stimulation that used to bring pleasure. The vaginal lining becomes thinner, less elastic, and drier. The physical changes in the vagina and surrounding area, including the urinary tract, are a result of lower estrogen levels.

Because of this, sex can become uncomfortable and even painful, which can certainly affect enjoyment and desire. Those changes can manifest themselves in specific ways: dryness and/or irritation of the vagina, itching and/or irritation of the outer genital area or vulva, and the need to urinate more.

I'll discuss urinary issues in a moment, but if you are experiencing pain in intercourse, it's important to have your doctor rule out a vaginal infection. If there's no infection and dryness is your main challenge, there are things you can do to minimize or even reverse this dryness.

First of all, know this: The physical and psychological aspects of hormone change may be putting a damper on romantic moments, but abstinence is *not* the answer. Not only does frequent lovemaking improve sleep, reduce stress, and help alleviate moodiness, but vaginal dryness is actually helped by regular sexual activity, which promotes circulation and lubrication. Also, there is some indication that sexual activity may stimulate estrogen production in the adrenal glands, which, in turn, helps to keep the vagina lubricated. In addition, the muscle contractions and increased blood flow that occur right before (and during) orgasm seem to "exercise" the vagina, helping it retain its "youthful" condition. Yet again, I marvel at God's miraculous design—that sexual intimacy rejuvenates and refreshes our entire well-being, in addition to rejuvenating and refreshing our relationship with our spouse!

To help with lubrication, if you've been looking for a truly compelling reason to drink more water—here it is, finally! Water is a great lubricant for your *entire* body. Get the eight 8-ounce glasses you need every day, and even more if you are having hot flashes on a regular basis.

Also, using a water-based lubricant, such as K-Y or Astroglide, may help during intercourse. These are better over-the-counter lubricants than oil-based petroleum jelly and can be used safely with condoms.

Vitamin E oil can also be used as a lubricant. This common vitamin supplement can also be used directly in the vagina to increase lubrication and soothe the vaginal lining. Women can buy vitamin E oil capsules sold in most drug stores, and crack open a capsule to get the oil. These should be used nightly for six weeks, then weekly or as needed.

Apart from intercourse, you may try using a lubricant that contains polycarbophil, such as Replens, daily for two weeks, then twice a week. These coat the surface of the vagina and moisturize the vaginal tissue.

You may require a longer period of foreplay before intercourse. The longer the foreplay, the longer your body will have to release its own natural lubricants.

If it's not discomfort but rather a lack of interest or energy for sex that you're experiencing, check with your doctor to be sure that there is not a treatable cause to your loss of sex drive. Beyond a potential decrease in testosterone (which can be supplemented), typical libido-busters are low thyroid levels, sleep disturbances, and certain medications (the pill, blood pressure lowering medications, and certain antidepressants like Zoloft and Prozac). But the most common is just pure and simple fatigue.

HONEY, I'M JUST TOO TIRED

You come to bed with one thought in mind—*sleep*. You turn to mumble "Good Night" and look into your prince's eyes, only to find them expressing an entirely different idea. The only thing you can manage to say is, "You've got to be kidding; do you have any idea how tired I am?"

Not "being in the mood" goes to an entirely new level in midlife. As we've already observed, women in midlife can find themselves facing changes and stresses in many areas of their life, which can lead to feelings of depression, stress, anxiety—and exhaustion. Somehow, sex is not on a woman's "to do" list when there is already too much to be done, too little time, and way too little energy. Since the brain is our primary erogenous zone, these feelings can undermine sexual desire.

At a different moment than bedtime (which is *not* the best time for open communication!), let your husband know how you are feeling and that it's not just about him. If there are things he can do differently to stimulate desire, let him know.

Also, it may be time to *make time* for romance. With most couples' busy lifestyles, it can be hard to give intimacy the time and attention it needs. You may need to actually "schedule" time together in order to create the space for emotional and physical closeness that may be missing. Remember? It's called *dating!* Counting on spontaneity in busy midlife is not a smart move when your love life is at stake.

Once the night is scheduled, plan for your romantic interludes—and prepare your body physically and mentally, the way an athlete prepares for an event. Seriously! If you're looking ahead to an evening "date for romance," take a power nap in the afternoon, be sure to hydrate with water, and power snack throughout the day to have the needed energy to make your night most enjoyable.

URINARY TRACT ISSUES, INFECTION, AND INCONTINENCE

Recurrent urinary tract infections or urinary stress incontinence (the loss of urine with coughing, sneezing, laughing, exercising, etc.) may occur because of the thinning of the estrogen-dependent lining of the outer urethra and because of blood sugar swings associated with perimenopause.

Severe cases may possibly require hormone replacement, at least for a temporary period, but urinary symptoms often can be resolved simply through Kegel exercises, which increase the blood flow to the area and help with stress incontinence. To do Kegels: Firmly tense the muscles around your vagina and anus, as if you are stopping the flow of urine. Hold for as long as you can, working up to eight to ten seconds, then slowly release the muscles and relax. Aim for ten to twenty-five repetitions two or three times a day.

Keeping your blood sugars stable—through eating well and often—along with positive water intake can prevent an overload to the system. Don't make the mistake of drinking less water in hopes of reducing urinary frequency. It is apt to backfire, for the resulting dehydration actually increases the concentration of urine, sounding a more urgent call! To first flush out the system, try to get eight ounces of water on the hour, every hour, for at least eight hours. Every time you urinate (which will be more often initially with more water!), be sure your bladder is completely emptied (helped by leaning forward while urinating).

To keep the urinary tract "environment" healthy, be sure you are getting sufficient vitamin C (go for oranges, red peppers, mangos, broccoli, and strawberries), try a six-ounce daily dose of 100 percent cranberry juice, and try a daily serving of freshly fruited yogurt (plain yogurt mixed with fresh fruit) with active cultures to help retain your balance of the "good" bacteria.

LOVE WELL, LOOK WELL!

Troubled by wrinkles around your eyes? Worried that your skin is sagging or those gray hairs are making you look your age? Have sex with your prince!

Making love three times a week can make you look ten years younger, claims a Scottish researcher—as does David Weeks, a clinical neurophysiologist at the Royal Edinburgh Hospital, whose ten-year study on the effects of sex on aging reveals some amazing results on youthful looks emerging from an active sex life.

With most of the participants in the study being forty-five to fifty-five years old, having sex an average of three times a week was found to be the second most important determinant of how young a person looked. Only physical activity proved more important than sex in keeping aging at bay. More frequent sex didn't seem to produce any added benefits, nor did casual sex with different partners or cheating on your spouse. "The sex doesn't work without a good relationship," say the researchers. "It works via a relationship that is very supportive and emphatic, in which both people are physically and emotionally compatible." Personally, I love this sort of statistical evidence that verifies the wisdom of living the way our Designer intended. It's fascinating!

In addition to the anti-aging impact on looks, sex also can burn fat and cause the brain to release endorphins, naturally occurring chemicals that act as painkillers and reduce anxiety. In men, sex seems to stimulate the release of growth hormones and testosterone, which strengthens bones and muscles. This probably holds true for women as well. In addition, in both men and women, research has shown, sex seems to prompt the release of substances that bolster the immune system.

Obviously, there are many other alternatives beyond romance for looking and feeling your youngest best. Read on!

MIRROR, MIRROR:
TAKING CARE OF YOUR SKIN,
HAIR, AND BONES

I have a question for you. Be honest: Is one of the more distressing parts of midlife your changing appearance? It certainly is for me, and for most of my friends. It's enough to have to deal with the body reshaping and necessary weight gain, but when skin begins to sag, spot, and wrinkle and once lustrous hair begins to dull—it's just too much for we lady boomers. And, of course, we are entirely too young for any of it!

To understand and turn it around, let's start with some basic science involved in changing skin. Generally somewhere around the mid-thirties, a tendency begins toward more dryness and the appearance of fine wrinkles. The collagen layer of our skin becomes thinner as we age and hormone levels fall; by midlife, we will have 20 percent less collagen than when we were twenty. In addition, our oil glands tend to decrease their secretions, resulting in a greater tendency toward dryness. Add to that package the years of sun exposure and damage, and we've got the formula for some definite changes in our skin and appearance.

To keep the issue confusing, often times in the heat of the hormonal transition, a woman may be besieged with what looks like teenage acne and oily skin. You may find yourself with the worst case of acne you've had since Junior Prom—your first breakout since high school—and it's because the hormone fluctuations are similar to puberty.

When it comes to hair, there may well be a connection between dwindling estrogen levels at menopause and thinning hair, though there is no conclusive data. It is important to check out possible thyroid dysfunction, but it is generally accepted that hair loss or excessive hair showing up in the wrong places is related to proportionally *higher* levels of the androgen hormones that goes along with the hormonal transition of midlife.

BEAUTY REALLY *IS* INSIDE OUT!

A wide variety of highly effective skin treatments are now available to help build collagen, resurface the skin, and prevent wrinkles. But having beautiful skin and hair is really an inside-out job. Adequate protein (eaten in a way that boosts its utilization), along with eating foods rich in phytoestrogens and essential fatty acids and getting adequate vitamins B, C, and E, also helps to build collagen and rejuvenate the skin. And then there's water!

Drink water! Drink water! Drink water! Water is one of the most effective pore purifiers around, and it is essential for lovely skin, hair, and nails! You will see a dramatic improvement if you'll just drink eight 8-ounce glasses each day; it's considered the original anti-aging, anti-wrinkle ingredient.

Power with protein. Getting enough protein is vital to be healthy—and lovely. You'll read more about it in chapter 19, but protein is the "new" you, working within to build collagen, protect the skin, and repair any damages. To get the best from protein's building power, eat smaller amounts of high quality protein-rich foods, evenly distributed through the day and protected with carbohydrate, to prevent the protein being cross-utilized for energy. Many women take in enough protein but not often enough to use it, so they lose it! An added benefit to eating protein often, and in a balanced way, is a stabilization of blood sugars and insulin production, which also curbs excess androgens, thereby helping skin and hair.

Make some of that protein fish, especially in the form of salmon, tuna, or swordfish, which are rich in omega–3 fats and are important for building healthy cell membranes everywhere in the body. You'll read more about how to accomplish this in chapter 23.

Up the ante on antioxidants. One of the benefits of the Hormone Balancing Plan is its inclusion of ten fruits or vegetables each day and the valuable antioxidants they provide. Many of their phytonutrients, such as lycopene in tomatoes, carotenes in sweet potatoes, or lutein in spinach, have been clinically proven to prevent and heal sun damage to the skin. As you'll soon read in chapter 20, the greater your variety of fruits and vegetables—and the brighter their color—the better it is for you and your skin.

Go with soy. Soy's phytoestrogens help strengthen collagen throughout the body—in facial skin, vaginal tissue, and your bones. One of the most common benefits women notice after several months of getting adequate soy into their diets is improvement in their skin tone, hair, and nails.

Focus on fiber. Nothing shows up faster on the skin than chronic constipation. Yet the stubborn midlife gut certainly can push you in that direction. You'll read more about this in the next chapter, but make sure you are getting enough fiber, particularly from whole grain carbohydrates like brown rice, oats, and whole wheat bread. They are also filled with vitamin B6, a vitamin used to treat hormonally induced skin problems.

One more time—water, water, water! For dry, itchy skin, moisturizers will also be a great help, especially when applied right out of the shower while your skin is still damp. This provides the best absorption. In the winter, try to keep heated houses well humidified and get into the sunlight whenever you can (protected with sunscreen, of course!).

BUILDING AND KEEPING STRONG BONES

It's fascinating to me that the very nutrients that build beautiful skin and hair are also at work building strong bones. I realize that bones seem stable as rock. In fact, however, they are made up of living cells—just like our skin and hair—that are constantly being broken down and replaced by new ones.

But when that breakdown accelerates and/or rebuilding slows, osteoporosis results—a serious issue for women approaching menopause. The National Osteoporosis Foundation recently released figures that show osteoporosis and low bone mass are a major public health threat for 55 percent of the U.S. population aged fifty and older. For women, the risk of death from osteoporosis is equivalent to that from breast cancer!

For many women, bone loss through the process of osteoporosis begins as early as age thirty, or perhaps even earlier. Because of chronic dieting, undereating, overexercising, poor nutrition, or eating disorders, many women do not reach the peak bone density they should when they are in their teens, twenties, and thirties. Thus, when a woman turns forty and her hormone levels begin to shift, the collagen matrix that forms the foundation of healthy bone may start to weaken, especially when a woman's nutrition and exercise regimens are lacking.

Osteoporosis is *not* a natural part of aging. As we get older, our bones do become less dense and weaker, but it is not normal to have porous and brittle bones that are susceptible to fracture. What can we do now to ward off this disease, which has been labeled a "silent killer" for women?

As you read in chapter 7, HRT was often prescribed in order to protect women against osteoporosis. Without doubt, estrogen helps maintain bone health. But there are safer alternative prescriptions and natural measures to be taken:

Fosamax: Fosamax, Actonel, and similar bisphosphonate medications are designed to prevent or treat osteoporosis; they slow bone thinning and increase thickness of the bones of the spine and hip. This reduces the risk of broken bones. The drugs are so successful that researchers are now looking at administering the drug through once-a-year intravenous infusions so women don't have to take pills every day.

Evista: A new class of designer estrogens are also prescribed to prevent and treat osteoporosis. Evista, also

Do Your Bones Need Help?

Bone densitometry is a fifteen-minute outpatient procedure that gauges bone strength. Most women should have the test at menopause to get a baseline, and even earlier if there are heightened risk factors. DXA or DEXA is the best test and is widely available; it's painless and quick and is done with very low radiation exposure. It measures the density of the hip and spine bones as well as total bone density. Insurance does not always cover this test; most policies are more apt to cover a test of the heel or wrist only, which is still a useful indicator of overall bone health.

known as raloxifene, was designed to selectively act as an estrogen on bone but not on breast tissue or the uterus (where estrogen can increase the risk of cancer). Evista has another plus—it has a favorable effect on cholesterol.

You can maintain the collagen matrix in your bones and also help rebuild healthy bone in a variety of natural ways, which include all of the skin and hair enrichers you've just read about, especially getting adequate phytoestrogens from foods such as soy. In addition, adequate calcium and exercise are the dynamic duo against bone loss, together with that well-balanced eating plan you've been reading about.

I've dedicated an entire chapter (chapter 24) to the building and stabilizing power of calcium. It's just that important. Women over the age of thirty-five should get about 1,500 mg a day of calcium, yet few women get the calcium we need, and the deficiencies started when we were teenagers. Dietary sources of calcium include fat-free milk, yogurt, and cheese.

Bones need other minerals, too—notably magnesium and phosphorus—but fortunately, plant sources of calcium also contain these other minerals. Here are four additional steps for building bone and preventing osteoporosis.

Get vitamin D. Vitamin D is critical for both absorbing the calcium you eat and for allowing the bones to remineralize with calcium. You can get all the vitamin D you need from thirty-two ounces of fortified milk, or from just twenty minutes of sunlight a day. (Skin makes vitamin D upon exposure to sunlight.) If neither of those two strategies is consistent for you, a supplement (about 400 IU) is vital.

Get moving. You'll also read more about the power of exercise in chapter 27, but as it relates specifically to osteoporosis, a well-developed exercise routine not only stimulates new bone growth but may also halt bone loss. It's one of the most natural remedies, and one that will also help maintain a woman's overall health.

Get at least thirty minutes of walking, weight lifting, or another weight-bearing exercise at least three times a week. Weight-bearing exercise is strongly recommended because it causes the body to generate more bone in the area taking on the added weight. It's been shown to increase bone density by as much as 2 to 8 percent per year. Brisk walking, jogging, stair climbing, tennis, dancing, hiking, and weight lifting are great choices for weight-bearing exercises.

Avoid high protein diets. Although getting enough protein is a good thing, getting too much *is not.* High protein diets have been shown to cause an increased loss of calcium from the bones along with an increased risk of kidney stone formation.

Get away from caffeine and sodas. More than 400 mg of caffeine a day (just two large mugs of drip coffee!) will cause your body to excrete calcium in your urine. Teas and coffees also contain oxalic acid, which can also interfere with calcium absorption, so be careful not to use to excess. In addition to containing caffeine, many sodas contain phosphoric acid, which significantly impairs calcium absorption and can lead to decreased bone density.

If you are looking for a replacement beverage—other than wonderful water—try green tea. It's available in a naturally decaffeinated form as well as regular. It is especially rich in phytohormones and antioxidants. Research has shown that women who drank green or black tea regularly had stronger bones than those in a control group who did not.

Interestingly, caffeine and soda are not only negatives to the strength of our bones, but they can also "disturb the peace" in our gastrointestinal tract. This is one more reason that water is the beverage perfectly created to hydrate our body—all of our days.

SOOTHING THE STUBBORN, ANGRY GUT

Burping and flatulence are not generally socially smiled-upon body sounds—or conversation topics! But why, oh why, does it happen in a crowded elevator? No one knows, but what brave (and somewhat quirky) researchers tell us is that the average woman passes gas fourteen times each day. It doesn't mean something's wrong; excess gas is just a natural by-product of a slower movement of food and waste through the system. However, it can be aggravated by hormonal imbalance and stress.

INCREASING GI DISTRESS

Serotonin regulates the gut as well as the brain. As a result, fluctuating estrogen levels can result in an increase in gastrointestinal distress: irritable bowel syndrome (or spastic colon), indigestion, bloating, distention—and gas. Excessive production of digestive acids in the stomach may cause painful burning and reflux after eating.

The muscles that propel foodstuffs along your gastrointestinal tract may begin to lose their elasticity and synchronicity somewhere in your forties, resulting in irritable bowel syndrome for about a sixth of all women. This condition is aggravated by stress. Over the long term, prolonged stress can disrupt the digestive system, irritating the large intestine and causing its muscular contractions to be spastic rather than smooth and wavelike. The abdomen becomes bloated and may cramp, along with rebelling against you with chronic constipation, diarrhea, or alternating periods of each. Sleep disturbances because of stress can further exacerbate irritable bowel syndrome.

Combine this bloating with PMS and perimenopausal mid-section weight gain, and you may wonder if you'll ever see flat abs again!

Gallstone formation is also more of a concern for a woman in midlife who is dealing with fluctuating estrogen levels, which promotes stone development. Add dieting, high-fat eating, and excessive weight gain to the pot, and you see why 20 percent of women in their forties develop gallstones or gallbladder inflammation.

The good news is that none of it — not irritable bowel, not constipation, not gallbladder distress — need be. All of it is pretty much remedied with a one-two punch: cutting fat and increasing fiber and thus lessening the aggravation factor of what you eat and the stress of your lifestyle.

CUT YOUR FAT AND DOUBLE YOUR FIBER

Fat intake signals a large amount of bile acid to be moved into the gastric area for digestion. This not only causes undue stress and strain on the gallbladder, the production site for bile, but it also causes irritation to the intestinal tract. All that bile being dumped into the more alkaline area causes intestinal spasms and inflammation. Cutting back on fat, particularly saturated fats, will make the healthy difference.

Fiber and water act together like a sponge in your digestive tract and help your food pass more easily. Soluble fiber, which is found in most fruits, some vegetables, and certain beans and grains, forms a bulky mass that keeps good motility and muscle tone and prevents diarrhea. Insoluble fiber, found in most vegetables, some fruits, and many breakfast cereals, can help prevent constipation. It is also associated with a reduction in diverticulosis, colon cancer, and other cancers.

You will automatically get more fiber by increasing your fruit and vegetable intake and putting focus on whole grains. You may also want to add flaxseed to your cereals or salads; they are not only loaded with fiber but also with beautifying omega–3s and phytoestrogens. Read more about flaxseed in chapter 23 and fiber in chapter 25.

In addition to adding in the fiber you need, here are some other tips to soothe the angry gut.

Drink water! Drink water! Drink water! Water activates the fiber you eat to produce a bulky watery mass that is more easily passed through the intestine. But, as an added twist, drink water *after* meals and snacks, not on an empty stomach, where even wonderful, simple water can cause a dumping of more acid into the intestinal area. Only sip water while eating and don't wash food down with any beverage, not even water. Avoid carbonated beverages.

Avoid tomato sauces and orange juice. Both of these cause even more relaxation of the gastrointestinal muscles (particularly the valve between the esophagus and the stomach), which allows more acid reflux (heartburn) to occur. Black pepper and chili powder are also irritants that can cause more acid to be secreted.

Avoid going long hours between meals. This also allows for acids to build up to explosive levels, with no food to neutralize it. Instead, follow one of the primary guidelines of the Hormone Balancing Plan: Eat well and eat often!

Chew your food and dine slowly. Mom was on to something here! Gulping food means gulping air, which ultimately looks for a noisy escape! The more slowly you eat, the less air you swallow and the better your food is broken down, and so the less likely you are to suffer from gas and bloating.

Be aware of the impact of the "gas producers." Vegetables such as melons, cabbage, cauliflower, corn, broccoli, brussels sprouts, iceberg lettuce, and legumes tend to produce gas. Yet (except for iceberg lettuce) many of these are the healthiest of foods, so they shouldn't be avoided altogether. However, if they affect you, you may not want to have large quantities all in the same meal. Eat them at different times and in smaller portions, or de-gas them by sprinkling on an enzyme mix like Beano.

Get moving! It helps to get your bowels on the move and prevents gas from getting — and staying — trapped. Walking can do wonders to relieve that bloated, gassy feeling.

Of course, exercise can do wonders in many parts of life, physically and emotionally. It serves as an offensive weapon in the war against stress, which calms the storm within and brings relief to gut pain — *and* head pain.

MENSTRUAL MIGRAINES

While the exact cause of perimenopausal migraines remains a mystery, most experts agree that changes in blood flow in and around the brain play an integral role. The pain and other symptoms of a migraine are thought to arise from alterations in blood flow and inflammation.

Migraines are headaches characterized by one-sided throbbing pain, nausea, and hypersensitivity to light and noise. They are three times more common among women than men. However, this gender gap is only present in adults; prepubescent girls and boys experience migraines at the same rate. It is estimated that six million American women have more frequent and intense migraines around the time of periods or during ovulation and that the headaches become more prevalent at the time of perimenopause, when hormones are in full swing. This, combined with the fact that migraines vary with pregnancy and menopause, has pointed the finger at fluctuating, imbalanced female sex hormones as a cause of the "menstrual migraine."

It usually comes just before your period, when both estrogen and progesterone levels fall dramatically. Stress and hormone triggers appear to cause electrical changes in the brain that lead to the opening and swelling of surrounding blood vessels. Estrogen fluctuations may turn on and off triggers that control these vessel changes, according to results of recent research that sheds new light on menstrual migraines.

Migraines occur when the arteries to the brain narrow and widen, a condition that activates nearby pain receptors. Drops in estrogen levels may trigger migraines by favoring this dilation and swelling of blood vessels surrounding the brain. The rising prostaglandin levels at your period that cause uterine contractions and menstrual cramps are the same chemicals involved in the menstrual migraine. Serotonin fluctuations also seem to be involved in this inflammatory process, as in just about every other perimenopausal symptom; it is generally believed that abnormally low levels of serotonin trigger these contractions.

NATURAL SOLUTIONS

Currently clinicians generally treat menstrual migraines the same as any other migraine. Over-the-counter pain relievers and anti-inflammatories help some women. For others, prescription drugs such as triptans are a better choice. Along with medication, doctors with a holistic bent help patients target and avoid headache triggers and reduce stress. Hormonal treatment is often ineffective and a last resort.

Natural solutions are the better bet and certainly should be the first choice.

Keep blood sugars stable. The right foods at the right time is the best prescription of all to avoid headaches and migraines. It's not just what you eat, but when; missing meals is a primary migraine trigger. The drop in serotonin that follows a drop in blood sugars is one of the strongest triggers to the vasoconstrictive action of vessels that leads to migraines.

Avoid refined carbohydrates and stimulants. Anything that triggers an adrenaline surge will also result in a drop in serotonin. Beyond sugar, sweets, and white, refined pastas and bread, other prime suspects are alcohol (especially red wine), caffeine, cocoa, and MSG.

Exercise. Exercise sets into motion the immensely positive cycle of relieving stress and releasing serotonin—a one-two punch against migraines.

Avoid fatty foods. Highly saturated and hydrogenated fatty foods are certainly a health hazard for conditions as varied as gallstones, breast cancer, and heart disease. But could a high-fat diet also be responsible for migraines? Maybe.

The elevated levels of free fatty acids in the blood that result from a high-fat diet can prompt a chain of events that culminate in the pounding headache characteristic of migraines. Fat in the bloodstream promotes changes in blood vessel walls and platelets, the cell-like particles in the blood. These changes appear to cause serotonin levels to fall, prompting a migraine.

Recent research shows that reducing fat can lower the frequency and duration of migraines. One study found that a reduction in dietary fat by an average of 60 percent was associated with a 71 percent drop in migraine frequency, a 66 percent decrease in headache intensity, a 74 percent decrease in the duration of the headache, and a 72 percent reduction in quantity of treatment medications.

Focus on smart fats. The key is balance and getting the *right* kind of fat—the essential fatty acids. We'll talk more about these in chapter 23, but for now know that omega-3s not only help lift depression but also work their magic on preventing migraines. Although a highly saturated and hydrogenated fat diet can trigger migraines, getting the right balance of essential fatty acids can prevent them. Because they supply the good prostaglandins, they help to strike the proper balance within the brain.

Go for the Bs, particularly riboflavin. Research has shown that foods that are especially high in riboflavin, a nutrient that helps the body to produce energy, are also effective in reducing migraine incidence.

In a study published in 2001 in the journal *Neurology*, researchers led by Dr. Jean Schoenen of the University of Liege compared the results of giving riboflavin or a placebo to fifty-five patients with chronic migraines. The researchers found that after a three-month period 15 percent of placebo recipients reported improvements in frequency and duration of migraines versus 59 percent of the riboflavin recipients.

Schoenen's team believes that riboflavin works by boosting a deficit in certain energy generators in the brain cells of some people with migraines. Regenerating this flagging energy system can prevent the mechanisms that trigger migraines, they said.

Riboflavin is found in a variety of foods, particularly whole grains and milk products. That bedtime snack of whole grain cereal and milk may be just what the headache doctor ordered!

MIDLIFE AND MIDSECTION WEIGHT GAIN: CRACKING THE FAT CELL CODE

Generally, the number one troubling perimenopausal symptom that women notice is a struggle with their weight; it's easier to gain, harder to lose. In your thirties, the first few pounds just mysteriously appear, no matter how you've eaten or how much you've exercised. In your mid-forties you may come to the horrific realization that your waist is two inches wider and your body is a full size larger. And by your early fifties, you are in a flat-out panic.

It's perimenopausal weight gain—and it's real.

It's also necessary, and for that reason it will be the most stubborn weight gain you'll ever experience. Like the weight gain of pregnancy, it has a divine purpose. For possibly the first time in your life, it's something to celebrate! The very pounds that used to be called "middle-age spread" are actually your body's genetic programming to help your transition through the hormonal change of midlife. Our fat cells are looking out for our menopausal well-being and are begging for you to cooperate.

What's frustrating is that the weight gain may come on at a much younger age than you would expect, go to places you don't like, and hang on much longer than you care for.

TELL ME AGAIN: WHY WEIGHT GAIN?

In midlife, as soon as your fat cells detect a slightly lower estrogen level, they come rushing to your aid to produce estrogen for you.

They increase their size, number, and ability to store fat. The fat cells in your abdominal region grow the largest because they are better equipped to produce estrogen than the fat cells in buttocks, hips, and thighs. This changes the weight issue for most women.

It's no longer about how much weight is being carried; in perimenopause, it's where the weight is being deposited. During the childbearing years, all excess weight seemed to go straight to hips and thighs to provide and protect for conception. Now it goes to the waist—and is most resistant to being burned because the body can better use it there.

The larger and more active your abdominal fat cells become, the more estrogen will be produced and the more benefits of hormone balance you will receive: fewer hot flashes, milder mood swings, less intense PMS, improved sleep, a reduced risk for osteoporosis, and an overall easier perimenopausal transition. A University of Pittsburgh study found that those women with the largest fat cells produced 40 percent more estrogen compared to those with the smallest ones. This is why heavier women have been reported to have less menopausal symptoms while thinner women have the most difficulty in and before menopause.

To become "bigger and better," the fat cells will attempt to put one and a half pounds of fat per year onto your perimenopausal body. That adds up to an average weight gain of about twelve pounds over the average of eight perimenopausal years. The thinnest women tend to gain the most weight during the transition to menopause, regardless of their caloric intake or exercise routine. A history of cyclical dieting (gaining and losing weight at least once a year) results in more fat deposition in the abdominal section. With our dieting ways, it's no wonder we are in the shape we're in!

If nothing else changes in a woman's lifestyle, this weight gain is accompanied by an increase in the amount of total body fat, especially in the upper body and primarily in the abdominal region. The body goes from the classic female pear shape to apple shape.

In addition, muscle mass declines, particularly if you do not use it. Women lose more than seven pounds of solid muscle mass per decade of adult life if they do not do enough physical activity—generally a loss of approximately a half pound per year.

The key words here that promote weight gain are "*if nothing in your lifestyle changes*," so that the hungry abdominal fat cells and the sacrificing muscle cells are allowed to go their own way. And go their own way they will; our midlife fat cells are just following an intricate set of instructions that is scripted into our very being. Of course, much *can* change, and hopefully will, which is why you are reading this book.

Some good news: The fat cell increase is not forever stuck in "store" mode. Once you stop menstruating and the hormonal balance is once again restored, your fat cells no longer are on a "seek and find" mission to accumulate more fat. The fat storage enzymes deactivate, and your fat cells actually shrink a bit in size.

But you don't have to wait that long to reclaim your body! My goal is to help you find your new natural healthy weight *now*, gain what you need for alleviating symptoms, prevent too much weight gain, and lose weight if you've already gained too much.

How much weight gain *is* too much? That is a difficult question to answer, because each one of us is unique and we are all starting from a different place.

Most studies show that for the majority of women, menopause alone will not cause excessive weight gain—not beyond what's needed for estrogen production—but overeating and underexercising will. It's a combined stew of cortisol surges, calorie overconsumption, and poor exercise habits that are all equally responsible for the added pounds. This is actually even *better* news! You can't do anything about the estrogen production transition and your body's response to it, but you can do much about overeating and too little exercise—right away!

Take heart! Excessive weight gain is not inevitable for women in midlife, nor is it impossible to control. If you have been gaining large amounts of weight or have been unable to lose it, it's probably because your hungry, hormonally charged fat cells are responding in a survival mode. Fighting them with a fad diet is *not* the answer; it only locks them into metabolic slowdown.

DIETING AND THE FAT CELL

The most serious grip of reality of all is this: The harder you try to lose weight through deprivation dieting, the more powerful your menopausal fat cells will become, and the more weight you will gain as fat. You may starve your body into weight loss, but it will be a loss of water and lean muscle mass, not the fat you so desire to lose. Muscle is easily lost during this time anyway, working in tandem with fat gain. Imbalanced dieting will simply take you from a larger rounded pear shape to a smaller rounded pear shape and ultimately, if dieting continues, a pumpkin shape. As a result, you will negatively influence your health and have exaggerated symptoms of perimenopause.

From puberty on, our metabolism slows 5 percent per decade. Thus, at forty-five, we're burning 15 percent fewer calories each day than we did at age fifteen. This drop in metabolism is partly the result of a decrease in muscle mass — primarily the result of lack of exercise — that reduces our ability to burn calories. If imbalanced dieting comes into the picture, the metabolism slows further still. With chronic stress added to the recipe, the resulting excess cortisol circulation adds even more fat storage to the outcome. As hormonal fluctuations and stress stir the bucket of food cravings and more calories are apt to come in, there's more to be stored.

That's why the only way to manage weight permanently is to forego dieting and begin to live in a new and natural way that unlocks the exit door to your fat cells so they start releasing fat again.

Getting your body working for you and shedding excess pounds is within your control. The key is learning and practicing strategies for staying fit and fueled that will get your body working for you with optimal fat-burning capability.

The Hormone Balancing Plan that follows in the next section is built around these strategies. It works to unlock your fat cells and restore the imbalances of your body and soul. The strategies are not vague or complex, nor are they startling discoveries. They are simply life keys to the real issues of hormone and weight management — keys to meeting real needs with real answers.

STOKE YOUR METABOLIC FIRE

It's not the calories taken in but the calories burned that count, and your metabolism makes all the difference. Remember, your metabolism is the chemical process that converts food to energy and is measured by how many calories you burn per minute for body functions—both voluntary activity and movement and automatic, involuntary functions like breathing, heartbeat, digestion, blood circulation, and hormone production. The largest amount of calories used (70 percent) are those burned to maintain this basic body functioning.

At a cellular level, our metabolism is activated with a balance of supply and demand. The cells demand a supply of optimum fuel and oxygen to make energy to supply the body systems, which in turn demand energy. While a calorie is indeed a calorie, your metabolism can increase or decrease (and thus burn or store those calories) depending on your eating patterns. The body is designed to slow itself down as a protective response to energy deficits. As a result, erratic eating patterns keep our metabolism locked into low gear, storing away every meal as if it were our last.

Think of your metabolism as a campfire that requires fuel to burn and air to fan the fire's flame. A campfire dies down during the night and must have wood added in the morning to begin burning brightly once more. Without being "stoked" with new fuel, the spark turns to ash, and there's nothing left to burn.

Similarly, your body awakens in the morning in a slowed-down state. If you don't "break the fast" with breakfast and continue to feed it through the day to meet your body's demand for energy and boost your metabolic system, your body turns to its own muscle mass (not fat!) for energy and slows down even more, conserving itself for a potentially long, starved state. Then, when the evening eating begins, most of that food will be stored as fat because the body isn't burning energy at a fast rate; the fire has gone out. The food you eat after long hours without is like dumping an armload of firewood on a dead fire. Sadly, there are many of us walking around with a lot of dead wood sitting atop our fires!

Regardless of the number of calories consumed when we do eat, the body can use only a small amount of energy, protein, and other nutrients quickly. The rest is thrown off as waste or stored as fat. Eating the American way robs the body of vital nutrients for the remaining twenty-four hours—until the next feeding frenzy. We not only go wrong in how much we eat or what we eat, but we also eat entirely too much at the wrong time. The vast majority of us get most of our calories after six o'clock in the evening—too much too late.

STARVING FOR NUTRITION

To burn the calories you consume—metabolize them into energy rather than store them as fat—nutrients are required. These vital nutrients are the vitamins, minerals, and phytochemicals found in foods. Certain nutrients are considered keys for metabolism because they act as catalysts for calorie burning. The B-complex vitamins, magnesium, and zinc are important examples. Also important is chromium, found in whole grains, which helps to transport glucose through the cell membranes so that it can be burned for energy. Iron is also vital because it delivers oxygen inside the cells, "fanning the flame" of calorie burning.

Many people may be getting plenty of calories but not enough of the nutrients to help metabolize those calories and activate fat-burning potential. Or, their metabolisms may be so slowed in response to the chronic stress in their lives that they cannot burn the calories effectively. Either way, there's a fat-storing crisis.

Living life in the fast lane (and often, the fast food lane!) means that food choices are often about convenience instead of nutrition. That translates to more than a junk food diet; it becomes more of a junk diet: lots of calories, lots of fat, lots of sodium, lots of sugar—all promising energy on the run. But it's energy that runs out and ends up slowing down, not speeding up, our metabolism.

The classic junk diet is notoriously low in the nutrients that provide for consistent, long-lasting energy. The vitamin and mineral value of our mealtime choices is at an all-time low. We are more apt to eat chips than potatoes, eat ketchup than tomatoes, and drink orange soda instead of orange juice. Because of these choices, most of us are deficient in the vitamins and minerals that would keep our metabolism working in high gear.

But we can make different choices. We can choose to eat well and eat often. To preserve muscle mass and burn fat while losing weight, your best bet is to eat balanced meals and snacks of whole carbohydrate and low-fat protein, evenly distributed throughout the day. This, in combination with eating an adequate amount of calories, is the most important step you can take to unleash your body's natural ability to lose weight. It prevents your hungry fat cells from locking down, sabotaging your weight-loss efforts.

To activate your metabolism and get your body working for you, you need to eat: Eat *early*, eat *often*, eat *balanced*, eat *lean*, and eat *bright*. Read more about this kind of eating in the next section—it's one of your first steps in the Hormone Balancing Plan and the first key to cracking the midlife fat cell code.

FANNING THE FIRE'S FLAME

Eating strategically is one of the best ways to increase your metabolism, and exercise is a close second. Yet research shows that most people with weight problems not only eat too much, too late, but they also exercise too little. Controlling your intake of food is not an alternative to exercise, nor is exercise an alternative to healthy eating. Both are important to total wellness.

Not only does exercise help you to better burn the calories you take in, but it also serves to build muscle mass. And that's another weight-control secret: To rev up your metabolism and burn fat, use—don't lose—your muscle. Building new muscle through strength training is one of the best ways to reverse the metabolic slowdown of midlife and stressful living. And since calories are burned primarily in your muscle, maintaining muscle mass is a key factor in helping maintain a healthful weight. The more lean muscle mass you can preserve, the bigger "engine" you'll have in which to burn calories.

Read more about the benefits of exercise in chapter 27.

TAMING YOUR CRAVINGS

Cravings and weight gain around your period are not figments of your perimenopausal imagination—or excuses; there are several bona fide links between women's hormonal hunger and fat metabolism. In fact, preliminary evidence suggests that you can actually take advantage of the mechanisms already in place in your molecular biology and that it may help you to manage your weight, shape, and appetite.

If out-of-control cravings have been driving you to the cookie jar every month since puberty, but now it's every day, here's what you can do to avoid packing on even more pounds over the long haul.

Eat often. Choose balanced meals and snacks. Get protein, such as an egg, lowfat cheese, or a cup of beans at every meal in order to help prevent wild cravings. Protein can give you a solid sense of satisfaction.

Get your calcium. Ideally, you need 1,200 to 1,500 mg a day from food and supplements. Although it may seem unrelated, research shows that adequate calcium works to reduce hormonally related cravings. In addition, new research shows that those on weight loss plans lose more weight if they are getting the calcium they need, as compared to those who aren't.

Exercise, no matter how bad you feel. The aerobic charge will boost your serotonin and dampen your appetite.

Sigh! There is no quick relief for midlife weight gain. There's nothing quick about turning this big ship—it turns slowly—but it *can* turn!

I want to help you reframe this important and fascinating period of your life and not be swept into despair over your body shape temporarily changing. As in pregnancy, you are not getting fat; your body is gaining necessary weight. A few extra pounds are a small price to pay for avoiding hot flashes, mood swings, sleep deprivation, and vaginitis.

Eating well in our forties, fifties, and beyond is less about being thin and more about giving us energy to step into our busy days and strengthening our immune system. The Hormone Balancing Plan that follows will help you accomplish just that. It will provide you with a week-by-week guide to embracing the principles you've been reading about and balancing your hormones. By putting focus onto establishing one new habit each week, you'll have a chance to embrace each one more fully—incorporating a new way of eating along with a new perspective on light and exercise into your new way of living.

Part 3

YOUR
12-WEEK PLAN
FOR HORMONE
BALANCE

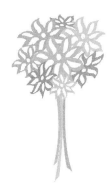

Tired, Wired, and Hungry?

Week
1

Here's what you've been looking for: a systematic, twelve-week plan to restore and maintain hormone balance, ushering in a sense of joy, peace, and purpose. Cycles of fatigue, depression, anxiety, or forgetfulness do not have to rule your days—or your nights!

Each week, you'll learn to activate new ways to keep the levels of "terrorist" stress hormones and brain chemicals from inching up into the danger zone and to encourage the levels of "peace-keeping, feel-good" hormones to rise—naturally.

With what you have read so far, you now recognize that there is a hormonal and brain chemical component to how you feel. That "Ah-ha" is the first step toward gaining renewed energy and vibrancy for life as you acknowledge that you are not simply getting old or losing your grip!

The next step is to decide what you *want* to change, internally and externally, to fully enjoy physical and spiritual vitality. With your new sense of the science behind the midlife body's changes and responses, you are ready to put a plan into action to reclaim balance in your hormones—for life.

HORMONES IN BALANCE WEEK-BY-WEEK GUIDE

As you now know, God's design of the human body incorporates an amazing ability to heal and repair itself on a daily basis. This capacity for wellness is scripted into every cell of your body; you only need to live in a way that nourishes it rather than hinders it.

Moreover, the secret to hormonal wellness and balance has also been placed within you: It is in your serotonin level. You can do your part to stabilize your brain chemistry and hormone production and to defuse the stress response by learning to make lifestyle choices that produce adequate serotonin and promote its function and circulation.

Almost deceptively simple, the Hormone Balancing Plan will address a number of complex systems all at once. The natural solutions I am suggesting are all about your daily choices for self-care: what and when you eat, what you drink, how you move, how often you get exposed to light, and whether you fill your spiritual, emotional, and physical needs with times of rest and replenishment. Use this step-by-step plan as if you and I were working together, sitting down face to face, meeting on a weekly basis.

As I do with my clients, we'll start with the basics. I want to help you take a look at how you live and eat, and to put together an action plan that will specifically target your needs and personal priorities. Using it, you will learn to read your own body and soul to see which factor is contributing to your symptoms—how to alleviate it and bring balance back into your life. You can revive your hormones and energy with simple strategies that can make the world of difference in midlife and beyond.

As we move through the process, you will also learn how the positive changes you are making will affect each of the biochemical imbalances we have been looking at. The lifestyle patterns you establish to feel great today are the very patterns that will help to protect you from the diseases of tomorrow—heart disease, osteoporosis, and cancer—and keep you feeling and looking younger longer.

I would encourage you to continue reading through to the finish of this book to get the big picture. Then come back and begin working through each of these action steps—week by week.

HORMONE BALANCING PLAN

1. Tired, wired, and hungry? Keep a journal of symptoms, eating and exercise patterns, life events, and feelings.

2. Learn that S-E-L-F is not a four-letter word; nurture your body with self-care, your soul through connecting with others, and your spirit through connecting with God.
3. Eat to defuse stress and stabilize blood chemistries. Eat whole foods early, often, and in balance.
4. Eat more fruits and vegetables for their anti-inflammatory and antiaging phytochemicals and brain-boosting vitamins and minerals.
5. Have a variety of phytoestrogen-rich foods.
6. Drink water—and a lot of it! Ideally, eight to ten 8-ounce glasses each day.
7. Focus on smart fats. Use extra-virgin olive oil as your main fat and increase your intake of omega–3s and other essential fatty acids, avoiding hydrogenated and trans-fatty acids.
8. Go for the calcium cure. Get plenty of calcium-rich foods.
9. Use whole grains for their phytochemical, vitamin, and mineral protectors and wealth of blood sugar stabilizing fiber.
10. Reduce your intake of stimulants: refined sugars, caffeine, and artificial sweeteners.
11. Embrace a well-rounded workout—strength training, cardiovascular work, and stretching—as your new way in midlife.
12. Get into the light, both physically and spiritually.

Do not be deceived by the simplicity of these steps. This is powerful medicine. Moreover, although these strategies are *simple*, they are *not easy*. Not easy, because each step to better living requires some measure of change, which is always difficult. Learning about soy foods, eating breakfast, strategically snacking through the day, trying new recipes, choosing whole grains, seeking and finding spiritual nourishment, developing replenishing relationships—all could be new and different to you. There is no magic pill that makes everything work all at once. Effort is required.

But trust me, it's worth it. Your investment into taking care of *you* will yield great rewards in your total being. You will start to feel better rapidly. As you come to understand how your blood sugar, serotonin, and hormone levels affect you, expect to become more and more excited about the hormonal balance you can achieve. Hormones going haywire is not a life sentence!

GETTING STARTED

In my experience, the best preparation for change is to identify your personal style for establishing new life patterns. Think about a time when you made a change in your life that really worked for you. How did you approach making that change? Do you prefer to do things all at once—diving into a pool head first—or do you take baby steps into the shallow end so that the process happens more slowly and you get accustomed to the temperature of the water?

How do you enjoy traveling? Do you like to have a plan or do you explore things more spontaneously? Must you know all the facts—have maps and guidebooks and well-orchestrated directions and schedules—or do you just take things on trust, as they come? Whatever you prefer, that's your own style for making change in your life, and the success of any plan is found in adapting it to fit your personal style. Although the Hormone Balancing Plan works much better if you take it slowly, week by week, it is important for you to start with who you are, even if it means doing everything at once.

However, it is my experience that you will have an easier time and be more successful if you don't try to "do it all." Instead, take it in sequence, step by step. Each step builds on the last. And each step belongs completely to you as you begin to make these changes, week by week.

FIND OUT JUST WHERE YOU ARE!

This is a great time to chart any symptoms you may be experiencing. Perimenopausal symptoms often fluctuate. You may develop new ones or find that those you now have suddenly get better, seemingly on their own. Because they are so impacted by your blood chemistries, symptoms can be aggravated or relieved by what is occurring on any given day in your life. However, knowing where you are at this particular moment will help you to get in tune with your body. Many of us keep such a relentlessly busy pace that it's easy to overlook or deny signs and symptoms, thinking it's just the stress of the day or the demands of the hour.

Pick up a simple spiral-bound notebook and use it to keep track for the next week, noting maladies that interfere most with your life. This symptoms diary will direct you. This is how you score: If your

- symptom is mild but present: score 1
- symptom is moderate and bothersome: score 2
- symptom is severe, disturbing life: score 3
- symptom is intolerable: score 4

As you review your own personal symptoms, you may quickly see certain ones that direly need your attention, such as hot flashes,

Symptoms Diary

Symptom	Score	Time of Day
Was your sleep disrupted last night with insomnia, frequent awakenings, or night sweats?		
Are you feeling depressed or "blue" for no apparent reason?		
Do you have any times of low energy or overall fatigue?		
Do you have any hot flashes or times of feeling too warm?		
Are you feeling restless, irritable, or anxious?		
Are there any moments when your heart is racing or pounding, even while resting or sitting?		
Are there any times of overwhelming brain fog or memory loss?		
Do you have any food cravings?		
Do you notice feeling bloated or fluid retensive?		
Do you have any sign of heartburn, gas, or an irritable bowel?		
Do you have any problems with frequent urination or urge to urinate?		
Is there any decreased interest in sex?		
Is there any sign of vaginal irritation?		
Does your hair or skin appear to be dry or your nails brittle?		
Are you fighting a headache or migraine?		
Are your joints achy?		

sleep disturbances, or violent mood swings. Put a red star by those. Others, like intermittent fuzzy thinking and sweet cravings, are more tolerable, but relief would be absolutely freeing.

After starring any intolerable symptoms, make a list of your desired goals to alleviate them. Express them in positive full sentences, such as: "I want to live free of hot flashes," or "I want to restfully sleep through the night and wake up feeling refreshed." You may want to transfer these goals to a three-by-five card to keep them ever before you throughout the weeks ahead.

Don't ever underestimate the value of making lifestyle choices that can improve your sleep, jump-start your energy, and restore a sense of peacefulness and contentment. You have the power to bring balance into a life that has been ruled by hurry and pressure. Later, we'll move on to address more lifelong concerns, but it will be alleviating immediate ones that will most motivate you to get on board with a new way of living.

In addition to charting any physical symptoms you may be experiencing, this is also the week to begin keeping a diary of everything you eat and drink, the time you eat, how you are feeling emotionally, and any exercise you may do. Before you make any changes in your lifestyle, you need to understand your body and how it is reacting to the choices you make. There is a blank Food-Feelings-and-Findings Journal on the following page. You may copy and use it, or just use it as a guide and keep track in a symptoms notebook or on your computer.

Although it may be tempting to skip this step, let me encourage you not to. It's really important. At this point, you may not know your own eating and lifestyle patterns and may not have more than a general sense of how you feel throughout the day. The journal helps you remember the details. It gives you a picture of the place from where you are starting. As you continue the Hormone Balancing Plan, you will enjoy being able to look back at your journal and see how far you have come.

Food, Feelings & Findings Journal

Date	Breakfast	Lunch	Dinner	Snacks	Exercise	Findings & Feelings

FOOD-FEELINGS-AND-FINDINGS JOURNAL: WHAT TO RECORD

- The date and time of your entry.
- List what you eat and drink, along with amounts. Be specific, even measuring amounts if need be. Record it as soon as you eat or drink something rather than waiting till the end of the day.
- Describe how you feel physically. Record the positive along with the negative. More than just "bad," write specific words like headache, stomach discomfort, muscle cramps or weakness, joint pain, fatigue, insomnia, hot flashes, chills, restlessness, shakiness, poor concentration or memory, pale, no appetite, or nausea. More than just "good," write if you notice stamina, high energy, restful sleep, focus, alertness, bright eyes, good color to your skin, increased libido, natural deep breathing, and natural hunger. Record these feelings whenever you notice them, not just when you eat, drink, or exercise.
- Describe how you feel emotionally. This may be more difficult; we are well trained in ignoring emotions. Although "bad" may be an easy word, try to find language to describe more vividly how you feel, such as anxious, bored, scared, mad, sad, depressed, scattered, restless, irritable, agitated, or hyper; rather than "good," try confident, excited, energized, humorous, happy, interested, focused, calm, relaxed, easy-going, or patient. As with physical symptoms, record these as you feel them.
- Pinpoint how connected and at peace you feel. This may be more difficult still.
- Describe your sense of spiritual health. Are you drawing closer to God through prayer, through his Word, through worship and fellowship? Does God seem near or far from you?

Your journal will teach you how to read yourself, giving you clues and symptoms that hint at the bigger picture. For this first week, as you keep track of how you are living each day, look for the areas that may be contributing to your symptoms. What patterns do you see with your eating, your exercise, your moods, and your feelings? For example, you may notice a distinctive energy drop in the thirty minutes after lunch each day, or a sudden (but regular) afternoon mood drop at 3:30 P.M. Or you may notice hot flashes more frequently on days that include Starbucks runs, or poor sleep after a bedtime bowl of frozen yogurt.

This process should be fun and informative—and free of negative judgment. This is not the time to beat yourself up over Krispy Kreme doughnuts or Big Macs; it's a time to simply record information that will help you see any connections between what you are eating, your exercise, and how you feel emotionally, spiritually, and physically.

At the end of the week, take a look at what you have written in the journal. Again, no criticism allowed—simply look at the facts, Ma'am!

Ask these questions:

- Do you eat regularly, at the same times each day?
- Do you eat between meals?
- Do you graze through the day, with no rhyme or reason?
- How long do you wait to eat when you are hungry?
- What kind of foods do you eat? Mostly carbohydrates or proteins?
- How many sweet foods do you eat in a given day?
- Do you use whole grains?
- Do you regularly eat soy foods?
- On average, how many servings of fruits and vegetables do you eat daily?
- Are you eating protein each time you eat?
- What kind of fats are you drawn to?
- How many caffeinated beverages are you using on a daily average?
- How much alcohol are you consuming?
- How much water do you drink on average each day?
- How many high calcium foods do you take in each day?
- How often do you exercise, and for what amount of time and intensity?
- How often do you get out in the sunshine?
- Are you sleeping through the night? How many hours on average?

You may not feel too great about your answers to these questions right now or even know why the questions (or your responses) matter in the whole scheme of health and well-being. Don't be discouraged — you will be learning! You'll also be changing many of these patterns for the better. And believe me, your results will be dramatically positive as you upgrade your habits and choices.

Once you find out just where you are, you can begin to work towards your destination.

HORMONE BALANCING ACTION STEPS — WEEK ONE

Keep a journal of symptoms, eating and exercise patterns, life events, and feelings.

- ✔ *Chart any symptoms you may be experiencing, using the guide on page 135.* Red star those that are interfering with your enjoyment of life — that is, those begging for immediate attention.

- ✔ *Keep a Food-Feelings-and-Findings Journal for this week,* recording what, when, and how much you eat, along with the specifics of any exercise you may do and whether it is indoors or out. Also, beyond what you are doing, record *how* you are doing — physically, emotionally, relationally, and spiritually, using the "Fuel Gauge" tool on the next page.

- ✔ *On day seven, assess your week, based on the questions just cited.* You now have a starting place.

- ✔ *Choose a buddy with whom you can talk through this hormone balancing process.* Set a time this week to get together and review your "trip" plans with her. Discuss your starting place and your destination!

- ✔ *Body-spirit balance step.* Spend at least thirty minutes this week doing something you enjoy — a warm bath, biking, reading, walking along the beach or lakeside, getting a massage (or dreaming of one!), and such. Pray aloud, chatting with God as you would a good and trusted friend. I thank God for leading me, guiding me—turning darkness into light, making the rough places smooth—and for not forsaking me. I often pray this Scripture:

I will lead the blind by ways they have not known, along unfamiliar paths I will guide them; I will turn the darkness into light before them and make the rough places smooth. These are the things I will do; I will not forsake them.

Isaiah 42:16

Fuel Gauge: Where Am I?

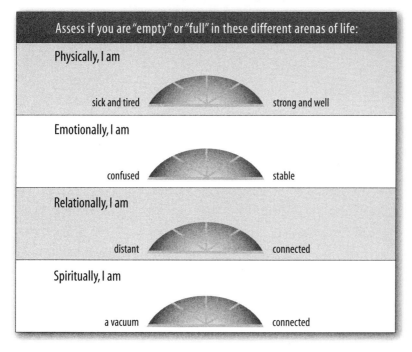

Assess if you are "empty" or "full" in these different arenas of life:

Physically, I am

sick and tired — strong and well

Emotionally, I am

confused — stable

Relationally, I am

distant — connected

Spiritually, I am

a vacuum — connected

Is S-E-L-F
a Four-Letter Word?

As women, we bear children and are caregivers of our household and the primary caretakers of our communities. It's no secret that we express ourselves differently than men do, giving words to our feelings and taking on an empathetic and nurturing role. And because we multitask so well, we can easily become run-down or ill—whether from simple fatigue, emotional imbalance, or a host of other ailments.

Such was the perfect descriptor for my client Christie—a working mom immersed in guilt about the time she spent away from home. When one child started struggling in school and her teenager was stopped for DUI, it triggered even more guilt. Then she and her husband entered into some difficult communication issues. Her aging mom was having more and more health problems, and Christie felt helpless in her ability to provide for her mother's emotional and physical care needs. Her brain read it all as life-threatening stress.

Christie stopped going to exercise classes at the Y and soon after stopped her morning quiet time and taking her daily walks—not feeling she could afford the time spent just "for her"; things were too out of control! And she was *so* tired; she couldn't get out of bed anyway. She started saying no to out-of-town business trips and any evening work activities, but then started fearing for her job, or at least her respected position within her company. She gave up meeting with her small group—women she had been meeting with for five years. She felt she just had to. She also determined to turn down any social engagements that didn't include the kids.

Stressed and Stuck

Getting stuck in the stress response can result from any daily challenge. But there are common outside forces that are unique to women "in the middle of life"; they are the currents that keep women trapped in the rip tide. They include:

1. divorce, death, or change in close relationships
2. child or career challenges
3. illness, either short-term or chronic
4. consuming caregiving
5. childhood traumas
6. perfectionism
7. chronic dieting

Feelings of sadness, worry, and anxiety suffocated any thoughts of self-care for Christie. She had lost her sense of balance and sank into a world of limitless giving. She was, in fact, damaging her important relationships — especially her spiritual life — and she knew it. Deep in her soul, Christie knew she was stuck in a vicious cycle of stress, but she didn't know what to do to get unstuck. She felt trapped and hopeless, and her hormones showed it. At thirty-nine she was battling PMS that was lasting up to twenty-six days a month, with little time to breathe in between. Her weight was up and her moods were down.

That's where she was when she walked in my door. I connected with this pained woman immediately, and her story hit me in the face with a sobering reminder. Her story affirmed a truth I know so well — that, like Christie, if we don't maintain the balance of self-care in our lives, our caregiving can become harmful as can the stress-stuck state in which we get trapped. Hormonal imbalance follows close behind.

How about you? Do you have times, like Christie, that you feel pulled apart and torn by conflicting demands of the many roles and responsibilities you're called on to fulfill? I surely have.

RIPPED APART AT THE SEAMS

As toddlers, both of my daughters loved Eeyore of Winnie the Pooh fame. One day, while one was playing peacefully with her beloved stuffed donkey, the other (who shall remain nameless!) decided *now* would be an excellent time for her to play with him. She grabbed one of his legs while her sister desperately clung to the other. Suddenly there was a ripping sound and a flurry of flying stuffing. Both began to cry, and there was poor Eeyore, lying on the floor split open, looking very sad and miserable indeed.

So again, the question: Do you ever feel like that donkey, pulled apart and torn by conflicting demands, literally coming apart at the seams?

- You promised your neglected mom a visit on Thursday night, and you find out your son is getting an award at school. Riiiipppp—you feel torn.
- You're on a deadline for a big project at work, and your daughter wakes up with strep throat and needs to see the doctor; you need to take her. Riiiipppp.
- There's an important group meeting you need to attend, but it will be the only night all week for you to see your husband. Riiiipppp.

The numerous tugs of roles and responsibilities are a huge burden of stress: commitments to employers, children, spouses, parents, friends, church, community, even yourself. It's hard to maintain a sense of wholeness in the midst of so much internal conflict. The energy requirement to do so wears on the soul, mind, and body. The "body wear" shows up in strong physical messages, many of them hormonal in nature. These messages are voices sounding a warning that you have been diverted from the path of self-care; these tangents manifest as physical and emotional "dis-eases."

FOOD FOR THOUGHT

Even though we may know certain elements of what to do to better care for ourselves, just doing it is not so easy. There's a huge difference between knowledge and action. If we acted on everything we know to do, every American would be eating breakfast and no one would be smoking. Alas, this is not the case.

It's not the case because *head* knowledge does not change lives. It never has and never will. It's only when we receive *revelation* knowledge into the heart that we are empowered to act on our new beliefs.

Oftentimes, what we most need revelation about is the truth of who we are and of our place of value. If you don't feel good about yourself, why treat yourself well? If you don't feel you deserve to feel good, why work toward that goal? If you don't believe it's possible for you to bring your hormones into balance, why try?

The reverse is also true. If we believe our body is fearfully and wonderfully made and designed to work for us, we will expect to be well. If we believe we are valuable, we will treat ourselves as such. A positive mental attitude is a vital spoke in the wheel of wellness and critical to hormonal and brain chemistry balance. In contrast, a negative state of mind saps our well-being and aims us toward just what we expect — the worst.

Focus is a strong factor in success. A winning athlete learns early in her career the importance of keeping her eye "on the ball," intently zeroing in on the goal. The prosperous businesswoman is one who sets goals and keeps her focus ever on them. It's a winning principle that we are drawn to what we set our eyes upon.

Yet this principle can work for the negative in life just as it can for good. Have you ever noticed how often automobile wrecks involve telephone poles? When a car is running off the road, there is much more open space to go toward than there are poles to hit. Yet they are what the driver sees, and they are what the driver hits.

If all we see is a menopausal nightmare before us and see nothing but a sinkhole of aging, hot flashes, weight gain, anxiety, and vaginal dryness, more than likely that is exactly what we will walk in. Because our eyes are set on problems and deficiencies, we will overlook times of feeling good, refuse to look toward help, and continue to propel ourselves into misery. Living in anxiety produces those very stress hormones that block serotonin and endorphins and further hormonal imbalance.

If we continually concentrate on what we don't have, we will more than likely get less of what we want. If we focus on what's wrong, we will never find what's right. Alternately, the people who are continuously rejoicing in what life gives them and are always looking for and expecting the best, lead active and fulfilling lives. Those who have the most beautiful lives are those who believe they can — and will. Choosing to keep a positive, optimistic attitude (i.e., the belief that you can take charge of your choices and influence your circumstances) protects you against sagging spirits, deficient serotonin, and hormonal imbalance by protecting you against the stress hormones that accompany hopelessness. There is *much more* to hormonal wellness than just caring for and nourishing your physical body. Those action steps actually begin with our thoughts and beliefs.

I believe we humans are both body and spirit; I also believe that both parts need to be nourished and cared for. To fully stabilize our hormones and to really enjoy life, we must have a way, and take the time, to recharge our physical batteries, to renew our spirits, and to connect with God, others, and ourselves. Otherwise, stress overtakes us; we get depleted, sick, and tired, and our body chemistries go haywire.

True wellness is not simply a product of physical well-being; it involves the interplay between body and spirit. We can nourish our inner lives and connect with God through reflection, prayer, and journaling. We can nurture our souls by forming deeper friendships and investing in time together. I've received the highest-quality fueling through participating in a life-giving church — one that celebrates, teaches, and loves God and people just like me.

The most significant way of contributing to our own good health is through the quality of our choices for self-care. It is one thing we have absolute control over in a life filled with a lack of control over so many other aspects.

WHAT *IS* SELF-CARE?

If we don't pay attention to the monthly siren call of PMS when our periods are regular, our symptoms seem to escalate as we get older. If we pay attention to the PMS-charged issues, we may see that these are only doorways to deeper issues and needs that have been ignored.

Constant "Pam-Questions": Have I accepted too much to do and yet have too little time to do it? Do I need more time off? Am I longing to be supported by my family? Do I feel grief for the lack of mothering time? Am I longing to be cherished by my husband? How do I find time to be with my widowed mother, who is growing older before my eyes? What do I do about missing face-time with friends? Am I not giving enough of me to my home, church, and community?

In the first half of our monthly menstrual cycle—the time when we are apt to feel upbeat and happy—we are also able to drown out our heart cries. But it doesn't mean the problems and needs aren't there. During PMS and perimenopause, these needs scream loudly; and when they are not acknowledged, they end up screaming louder and louder.

I started coaching Kathy for hormone balancing when she was forty-three, with two teenagers and two children under five. She first thought she was dealing with postpartum depression, combined with her second round of parenting in her late thirties. ("I'm just too old for this!" was her theme song.) However, hormone studies showed something different, that although a mother of young children, Kathy was close to menopause. She was still having periods, but erratic ones.

She had a rather funny view of it all, writing this on her initial assessment:

> This time of "hormones-gone-mad" is giving me so much perspective. It made me cry last week when I got caught in road construction traffic. I could clearly see that hold-up as a deliberate plot by the Department of Transportation to make me late for my appointment. It made me pick a fight with my daughter over a really critical issue—she left her flipflops by the phone. I suddenly saw her sloppiness as a sign of my improper mothering. And my husband! He didn't put out the recycle bin early enough to catch the truck, which was clearly a sign that I'm not valuable enough to help and that our relationship is headed for the brink.
>
> Then POOF! My period finally arrived, and I woke up to a beautiful world. Gone was the desire to get a divorce, put my kids up for adoption, and quit my job. I immediately stopped obsessing on getting lost in Europe. In fact—compared to the week before—I love my life!
>
> And so it's going these days—month after month. HELP!

Kathy loved and cared for her family, but she was a woman desperate for self-care, and her PMS attacks were not going to let her ignore it any longer. Like her, many women find that giving attention to their changing body is forced on them through the heightened PMS that blossoms into perimenopause, leaving them with the desire to pay more attention to its care. We are indeed living on and living longer, and we might as well live in the healthiest, most vital body possible.

If fulfilling this desire to "treat yourself well" seems out of reach, be encouraged by the truth that we can all find refuge even without escaping to a desert island!

I KNOW, I KNOW — IT TAKES TIME!

So you feel as if there's no time for you? It doesn't have to be job-related time pressure. It may be family or even ministry; the demands are nonetheless exhaustive. You probably know you should spend more quality time on yourself but just thinking about how to fit it in gives you a migraine. Just a moment alone seems an elusive dream!

Many of us push ourselves into prolonged periods of exertion without adequate periods of rest and replenishment — living long days with barely time for a bathroom break, and definitely no time for lunch. Some go months, even years, without a vacation or a relaxing weekend. No wonder we get run down and feel robbed of the joy and peace we so desire.

This breakneck pace not only inflates your stress level but also takes a hefty toll on your hormones, metabolism, and quality of life. And it prevents you from spiritually connecting and receiving.

If you are approaching meltdown, the best thing to do, ironically, is nothing at all — even if for just a moment. You were created by God with a need to rest, to recreate, to reflect, and to be regenerated. Without proper rest, you can become burned-out, bitter, sick, and tired.

LACK OF REST DANGER SIGNS

- grouchiness
- forgetfulness
- indecisiveness
- lack of creativity
- lack of humor
- lack of spontaneity

If you can first acknowledge and affirm your need for rest, then you can clear some time and find a quiet retreat — daily. You can unplug the phone, dim the lights, draw a bath—and relax. Taking time for replenishment is really a lifestyle. It makes a statement that "you deserve a break today."

Here are some ways to achieve a wiser, saner, and hormonally balanced you.

Chill out! Countless studies have documented the benefits of chilling out. Anything that relieves stress also boosts physical, spiritual, and emotional energy and becomes a metabolic booster. Fatigue disappears; backaches vanish; colds and flu are kept at bay; blood pressure drops; and chronic conditions—such as migraines, irritable bowel syndrome, insomnia, even acne—improve.

Sure, it used to be a little easier to get a break. Ten years ago, most stores were not open on Sundays. Now, Sunday is a day for shopping; the notion of the Sabbath being a day of rest has disappeared. You can go to the all-night supermarket and get your entire week's food at 3:00 A.M. And holidays—even those like Labor Day and New Year's Day—are a merchant's delight, a time for some of the biggest clearance sales of the year.

Trim your calendar. Just because you *can* do everything doesn't mean that you *must* do everything. Ruthlessly cross out unnecessary events on your calendar. Time pressure is a *huge* hormone wrecker.

Research tells us that although we feel more rushed and harried than we did twenty or thirty years ago, we actually have more free time than we used to. We just feel pressured to do more because of our super-speedy culture. E-mail, laptops, and cell phones create the illusion that we can, and should, be busy and productive every minute of the day.

While you cannot always stop responsibilities from piling up, you can pick what requires immediate attention and what can be put on the back burner. So go ahead, cancel some social events and not-so-vital work commitments and do exactly what you want. It will energize you beyond words and remove a major logjam to your hormone balance.

Make a date with yourself. At least once a week, carve out one hour (or longer) for your own—an hour in which you have nothing to do. Plan ahead on when that hour will be, but don't plan what you'll do; otherwise, it will become one more thing on your to-do list.

I actually try to spend one day a week in "rest," whether it's Sunday or another day. I need a consistent weekly withdrawal to do replenishing activities. A day of rest for me means a day of activities that personally revitalize me. It may mean reading novels, taking leisurely walks, napping, enjoying friends, window shopping, or just sitting, daydreaming, and writing. When I write, I am writing about me — what I'm experiencing, what I'm feeling, where I'm going — similar to the accompanying "You Are the Project; Life Is the Subject."

For some people, this kind of activity will provoke anxiety. For them to relax and be replenished, they need to be skydiving, sailing, or competing in a triathalon! And that's fine! "Relaxing" means different things to different people. Just switching to a different activity, even if it's physically strenuous, can revive you.

Studies have shown that curiosity increases our performance capability. When devoid of stimulation, people become disorganized, lose their intellectual ability to concentrate, and decline in coordination. So read a new book, paint your masterpiece, and seek out new situations, work opportunities, and challenges. We are stimulus-hungry beings, and denying our nature can lead to inertia and listlessness.

Start your day with a time of replenishment. Many of us

You Are the Project; Life Is the Subject

A project notebook can help give some form to your time of change. Keep a small jotter that you can carry with you and write down thoughts, quotes, things you might like to try, areas you might want to explore — in the world and in yourself.

Pay attention to other women: What are they doing? How are they dealing with this transition? Pay attention to yourself: What gets you passionate? What gets your juices going? What makes you uncomfortable?

Writing about stressful events not only may help improve your memory, but it also is a good way to take care of your emotional health. Writing about your worries may help relieve stress. This, in turn, causes the body to produce less cortisol, that major stress hormone that triggers hormone imbalance. Express your worries in a journal, in a letter to family, or in an email to a good friend.

Write about what is going on and how you are proceeding on new paths. It can help you recognize the cycle of change. Record your feelings, reactions, and dreams. Read them for internal clues to what is happening. You may see that you already know what your next step will be.

have learned the power of starting the morning with a quiet time of reflection and spiritual connection with God. This is a daily part of my life because I know that I could be doing nothing more important, and that it is the only way to start my day with strength. It is a moment of stillness in the midst of my busyness to reflect on what my source of strength really is, who I really am, and that nothing, *nothing*, is worth being robbed of the joy of life. Starting my day with quiet reflection is like the warm-up for my exercise—a time to stretch spiritually and get my soul circulating.

Let me give you a picture of my most typical day. I get up and eat breakfast (body fuel) while reading Scripture (soul fuel). Then, I exercise. While exercising, I'm also reflecting—not just going through a mental checklist and to-do list, but taking a step beyond to look at the "why" of my life: What's my passion? What is the purpose to which I've been called? Am I in step with God's plan for me? I sometimes ask myself why am I doing all these things and why am I spinning so many plates? *Oftentimes I need to focus more on what I need to say no to more than on what to say yes to.* I pray aloud as I walk; sometimes I put familiar Scriptures to tunes and sing them (guaranteed to get strange looks from the neighbors putting out the trash or walking their dogs!).

After this time of listening and reflecting, journaling is the way for me to get my thoughts and feelings into a place where I can take action. Writing down what's inside of me is a ten-minute investment that yields huge dividends. I journal my prayers, and I journal the answers and encouragement that I receive. It's my time to give my cares to God—to let go of what I don't want, don't use, and don't need. I leave this time uplifted and drawn to new challenges because I'm not struggling to carry the old.

If the idea of a quiet time is new to you, you might think of it as a Body-Spirit Balance Step. Throughout the weeks ahead, I'll be giving you ideas and encouragement for action steps you can take to develop new habits of caring for yourself. It's a most vital aspect of the Hormone Balancing Plan—and peace.

Take a power nap—a snooze you can use! A power nap can also be refreshing, relaxing your body, clearing your mind, improving your mood, and boosting your energy levels. Studies show that you don't really have to sleep to get the rejuvenation you need—just shut the door, unplug the phone, turn off the lights, and close your eyes. Rest and be replenished. Then get up and have a power snack (more on that later!). Stretch or take a quick walk at the end of your break to rejuvenate yourself for the work at hand.

If you choose to nap, make it short and sweet. Don't tell toddlers this, but a fifteen- to twenty-minute nap seems to be ideal for the maximum energy boost. You can stretch it a few extra minutes, but don't go over an hour. Napping too long can be counterproductive; long naps allow you to enter into the deeper delta-type sleep, causing a groggy, disoriented state when you wake that takes a long time to snap out of. If you seem to need more than an hour's nap in the afternoon, you're probably not getting enough sleep at night.

End your day with a time of relaxation. A while back, I began to end my day with a time to unwind. This is difficult for me; I have to tell myself more than once that there is nothing more I should be doing. I then enjoy some of my favorite things that don't seem very productive in the scheme of life, yet I know are vital to recharge my energy: reading travel magazines, listening to favorite music, taking a bath, whatever.

Again, it doesn't come naturally for me, because I'm a "doer" by nature. The first one up in our household, I go nonstop till the sun goes down and beyond. Even my "breaks" have often been purposeful: planning, researching, meeting with a small group. I have laughed for many years about being a "human doing" rather than a "human being," but only in recent years have I realized it's not something to laugh about. Ending my day with a time just to "be" reaffirms in my own mind that I am only human — and that's more than enough!

Does all this sound more like the ideal than reality? It needn't be. This is a great time to carve out our personal hours of renewal because living in contemporary society has made our need desperate. With determination and a little creativity, anyone can make time for refreshing.

Something happens to me when I choose to relax and be replenished. I return to what I was created to be. With time invested in recharging, I can review how I'm normally spending my time and reevaluate according to the purposes that have been placed in my heart. Otherwise, I stay too busy for issues of the soul.

After a time of quiet, I can look at my life demands more clearly, and I am more equipped to choose the perspective from which I am viewing them. This requires that I "stop, look, and listen." Otherwise, I become engulfed in what's wrong in my life and feel unable to see any light, any hope.

And this is why I deem nurturing your body and spirit as a vital second step in the Hormone Balancing Plan. It is the foundation from which you can make other lifestyle enhancements; by renewing your mind, you will be transformed. It's a promise!

HORMONE BALANCING ACTION STEPS—WEEK TWO

Enter into a new dimension of self-care. Set a high priority for times of replenishment and reflection, cultivating a positive perspective and nurturing both body and spirit.

- ✔ *Refer to the sample meal plans on pages 171–73.* These plans give examples of how to fuel your body with the right foods at the right time.

- ✔ *Take a hard look at your time use; is there time for a body-spirit balance step?* Are there moments of refreshing and relaxation—just for you and your Creator? This week, find at least a one-hour block of time—canceling something if need be—to schedule a time of replenishment. Choose to do an activity that uniquely nourishes *your* emotions and spirit.

- ✔ *Make a list of friends in whose company you feel more alive, happy, and optimistic.* Pick one with whom to spend some time with this week.

- ✔ *Take a walk.* Really, just for ten minutes each day. Even if you are already exercising, take a walk in addition. It has nothing to do with your eating choices but everything to do with treating yourself well.

✔ *Just breathe.* Slowly, deeply, from the diaphragm. "Take five" each day—five minutes to "practice" mindful breathing. Breathe in through the nostrils to a count of four, and breathe out from the mouth to another count of four. Breathe out stress, breathe in peace.

✔ *Continue to write in your Food-Feelings-and-Findings Journal.* This week, dedicate ten minutes each day to recording your thoughts and prayers from your time of replenishing and reflection. It just may be the start to journaling you've been seeking! A good beginning can be the promise found in God's Word:

Do not conform any longer to the pattern of this world, but be transformed by the renewing of your mind. Then you will be able to test and approve what God's will is—his good, pleasing and perfect will.

Romans 12:2

OFF THE ROLLER COASTER OF FATIGUE, STRESS, AND SWEET CRAVINGS: EAT WELL, EAT OFTEN

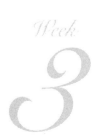

Strategic eating is the first line of defense in the midlife war on your brain and body. Because your brain is in need of certain nutrients found in everyday foods, eating well is the natural solution for establishing body peace. It may surprise you to find out that your body could literally be *starved* for serotonin. It may also surprise you to learn that although nutrition plays a key role, developing a plan to bring balance to your hormones isn't about going on a diet. Instead, it's a life plan, one that you will be designing for yourself, but not *by* yourself. You will learn which foods contribute to your overall health and when it is best to eat them; for hormone wellness, *when* you eat is almost as important as *what* you eat.

Debbie is a recently remarried mom of six children. She is forty-four years old, her own daughters are eleven and thirteen, her new husband's children are twelve, eight, and five—and the surprise one is just fourteen months. She comes to see me for a simple reason: She's basically out of her mind.

With all signs pointing to early menopause, Debbie started on Prempro (estrogen and progesterone replacement) before she married Mike. At their wedding reception, she actually credited HRT as God's blessing that allowed enough physical and emotional stabilization that she could lift up her eyes to see the new love of her life. Thinking she was long past fertility, she didn't use birth control or go for a pregnancy test until she was already four months along. The test revealed Debbie to be very pregnant, quite surprised, and yet absolutely thrilled and in awe of the new creation growing within her, the fruit of the miracle of the new relationship she had been blessed with.

But now, that little fruit is making her a little nuts. Sleep deprived and malnourished, joy is not abounding. Her standard answer to "How are you?" is "As good as a tired, fat, and forty-something woman with eight hot flashes a day, a migraine that doesn't stop, and a belly that begs the question 'When are you due?' can be." Our first meeting is not a delightful one.

Her day starts early, and she wakes up tired. The alarm jolts her out of bed at 5:30, and the morning routine gets started: kids out of bed and out the door, breakfast for them—no time for her. As an accountant, her day is full and mentally taxing; eating is catch and catch can: "I do errands at lunch time but try to at least grab a Chik-Fil-A. But sometimes I get back to the office and realize I never got lunch, so chocolate cookies have to do!" And by 5:00 P.M., the time she wants to be the best for the people she loves, she is exhausted, cranky, and craving sweets. But then, her work really begins! By 8:30, she's apt to be on the couch in a coma—only awakening due to a hot flash. Debbie's "I need help!" plea may sound like your own.

I'D RATHER BE ... ANYWHERE BUT HERE!

As I have noted about research into other cultures, not all women experience menopause the same way. The Japanese, for example, do not even have a word for "hot flashes," indicating that they do not experience them as Western women do. Japanese women also experience menopause much later, around an average age of fifty-five rather than our fifty-one. They also have one-sixth the rate of breast cancer than the United States. But when Japanese women move to the West and adopt the American diet, they develop hormone maladies and health issues similar to ours. It is not a genetic factor protecting Japanese women, but more likely it is their lifestyle—specifically their dietary choices—that power them with abundant nutrient solutions.

In our frenzied, convenience-based eating habits, we have moved away from the very functional foods that have served women well for millennia, and we are paying a price. Yet, by adopting these highly beneficial—and delicious—food choices as your own, you can provide for the alleviation of many midlife maladies. If there was ever a time to pay attention to what you eat, now is that time.

The basic plan for hormonal balance? You've picked up on it already: It's a meal plan that's loaded with fresh fruits and vegetables, whole grains, low-fat dairy products, healthy oils and seeds, legumes, lean meats, seafood, and fish—timed and balanced evenly throughout the day to stabilize blood sugars and nourish your body.

Ideally, your eating plan should be based on the cornerstones of freshness and variety. It should cover all the nutritional bases, supplying all of your needs for energy and wellness and minimize the intake of any harmful elements in food. It should be built from the most unprocessed foods possible with a healthy balance of whole carbohydrates and lean proteins and an abundance of brightly colored fruits and vegetables. Because ample calories are vital to getting ample energy and hormonal balance, your daily eating should supply at least 1,500 calories a day eaten in balanced, proportioned mini-meals throughout your waking hours. Most of all, it should provide you with great tasting food that is a pleasure to eat!

Ideal? Maybe. Reality? Probably not. Yet, let's take a closer look at what's really important and why.

THE HUNGRY BRAIN

It may surprise you to learn that your brain is a glutton for the sweet stuff in your blood, namely, *glucose*, its only fuel source. If the tank is running low, the brain functions at a deficit. Fatigue, mood swings, headaches, anxiety, and poor short-term memory are the early symptoms of insufficient blood glucose levels. Not eating, or not eating the right food, starves the brain, and the resulting drop in blood sugar sends you into "brain alert." Surges of stress chemicals follow. This spells bad news for a midlife body that's already stressed and hormonally challenged; it results in a wired-but-tired feeling, interrupts sleep, and fans the fire of hot flashes.

The solution is to satisfy the hungry brain with the right food, at the right time, and in the right balance. It's the ideal way to keep your brain chemicals, like serotonin, in balance all the time. However, supplying the brain with proper levels of blood sugars does not mean eating sugars and sweets; just the opposite is so. As you will later learn, the best form of brain food is *whole* foods.

Your nerve cells depend on a normal range of blood sugar—not too much, not too little—to function optimally. Nothing is more critical to your well-being. The required level is largely determined by what you eat and when.

THE MAKING OF SEROTONIN

When you eat food, your digestive system breaks it down into individual nutrients, like glucose and amino acids, to be absorbed into your bloodstream. Once absorbed, specific nutrients cross into the brain to speed the production of mood-enhancing neurotransmitters like serotonin. Nerve cells can't survive and thrive without adequate blood sugar; it's our body's original mood elevator and smart drug. The proper blood sugars can take away the blues and soothe irritability; it can perk up memory and concentration. However, deficiencies of blood glucose can cause the brain to malfunction and throw your body out of balance, and high levels can be just as detrimental. Worse yet, wide fluctuations in blood sugars flood your body with stress hormones, blocking estrogen and progesterone supply and effectiveness.

When our blood sugars are up and even but not too high, our brain is being fueled to make serotonin. We are brimming with energy and vitality, and our appetite is in control. When the levels are bouncing widely and wildly, our brain is being starved and energy, mood, memory, clarity of thought, and overall performance are apt to rise and fall along with blood sugars.

Blood sugar levels normally crest and fall every three to four hours, and even more often and intensely when your body is stuck in the stress response. If you've starved all day, the drop in sugars will be a "free fall," leaving you weak, sleepy, dizzy, *and* hungry. As sugars fall, so will your sense of well-being, energy level, concentration, and ability to handle stress. Your body will need about half an hour to convert what you eat to energy, so waiting until you're cranky and starving doesn't immediately rectify the situation.

There's one thing that doesn't fall with blood sugars, and that's your appetite. As the blood sugars crash, the body responds by sending a chemical signal to the brain's appetite control center, demanding to be fed. Your cells are screaming for a quick energy source — not broccoli or cauliflower, but chocolate, chips, or Reese's peanut butter cups!

Too much sugar and refined carbohydrates is a drain on anyone's energy metabolism and a serious one for people with sensitive blood sugar responses. Once a person who is sensitive to the rises and falls in blood sugar has eaten, her blood sugar rises quickly — very quickly if she has consumed a refined carbohydrate that is fast-released into the bloodstream as glucose. And that's the problem: What comes up quickly will quickly come down. You'll read more about these fast-release foods in chapter 26.

That's why a major secret of hormone balance is to eat in ways that give your brain cells steady access to desirable levels of blood sugars. This means eating well — and eating often. A poorly nourished brain is not able to withstand the whipsaw of hormone shifts, but a mind that is fit and fueled has a hormone advantage. In fact, by adjusting what you eat, you can deal with the three key issues of perimenopausal symptoms all at once: You can stabilize your blood sugar level, you can boost your serotonin levels, and you can minimize hormonal fluctuations. You don't have to cope with three different treatments, three different medication dosages, or complex instructions. You don't even have to try to understand it all. By making simple food changes, your body chemistry and brain chemistry will come into balance. You will feel energetic, optimistic, grounded, competent, easygoing, and connected.

Hormone Wellness
Eat Right Prescription

Eat early: Breakfast is the most important meal of the day!

Eat often: Power meals or power snacks every 2½ to 3 hours.

Eat balanced: Whole carbohydrates and lean proteins every time.

Eat whole foods: Choose food over supplements.

Make breakfast a must. Getting the day off to a good start is the single greatest factor in stabilizing hormone and appetite levels throughout the day. Breakfast takes your body out of its morning resting metabolic state and serotonin deficit, balancing your blood sugars and boosting both energy and hormone-producing capability.

Many women who come to see me initially balk at eating breakfast daily. "I can't face food in the morning," they say. "Why should I eat if I don't feel hungry?" The answer is that all bodies need food after a period of fasting, such as the time from dinner to breakfast. If you don't feel hungry in the morning, it's a sign that your body's chemical balance is awry and your hunger thermostat is not working properly. There is only one way to fix it, and that's establishing a focused routine of eating, starting with breakfast.

Once you begin to eat breakfast regularly, you *will* begin to feel hungry in the morning; this is a good sign! It means your body is starting to regain its chemical balance. You may also find you feel much better right away.

To get the most out of breakfast, eat soon after you get up (within the first half hour of arising). Have three different foods for breakfast: a quick, energy-starting simple carbohydrate (fruit), a long-lasting whole grain complex carbohydrate (grains, cereals, bread, or muffins), and a power-building protein (dairy, egg, soy, or meat). This good-for-you balance will allow a slow and steady release of glucose into your bloodstream to feed your brain and muscles with vital energy. Selecting whole foods rather than a Danish and coffee also gives your body the vitamins and minerals it needs to transform the energy nutrients into usable fuel. See the accompanying sidebar for some sensational breakfasts, many that you can do on the run!

Don't be afraid to experiment with breakfast ideas; your mom isn't in charge of

Balancing Breakfast Recipes

your breakfasts anymore! If you can face pizza, chili, or tuna fish better than eggs or cereal, go for it. Just make sure that you have it, have it soon, and have it balanced.

Have mini-meals. Instead of eating three big meals a day plus random snacks, eat five or six smaller, balanced meals spaced evenly throughout your day. Once you get the day started with breakfast, the goal is to keep your metabolic system and blood chemistries working for you. To prevent your blood sugars from dropping and to keep your metabolic rate and serotonin levels high, you need food distributed evenly throughout the day.

Going many hours between meals causes the body to slow down metabolically so that the next meal is perceived as an overload. Even if the meal is balanced and healthy, the nutrients cannot be used optimally. Again, it's too much too late. The lowered blood sugar will leave you sleepy and craving sweets—both effects of high cortisol and lowered levels of serotonin. And the high cortisol will block your hormone production and effectiveness. Instead, keep your energy and concentration up and cravings down throughout your day by eating small amounts more often.

Great Breakfast Ideas

- Oatmeal cooked in skim or soy milk, with cinnamon, vanilla, and golden raisins
- Low-fat or fat-free cottage or ricotta cheese with sliced berries and whole grain cereal
- Two-egg-white omelet with salsa and whole grain toast or whole wheat tortilla
- Open-faced toasted cheese sandwich with sliced apples or pears
- Yogurt parfait with berries and whole grain cereal
- Smoked salmon on toast with sliced tomatoes
- Whole grain toast with peanut butter (or soy butter) and banana
- Power shake with skim or soy milk, frozen berries, vanilla, and flaxseed
- Breakfast burrito with scrambled eggs and salsa
- Whole wheat French toast topped with yogurt and fruit
- Black beans and brown rice with grated cheese and salsa
- Peanut or soynut butter and all fruit jam tortilla roll-up
- Pita pizza (pita with tomato sauce and mozzarella, top browned)

I call this "power snacking"—eating the right amounts of the right foods at regular intervals—and it's an important component of hormone balance. Power snacking is a valuable tool for equalizing brain chemistries because it gives an immediate supply to meet the demand. Each meal should supply you with at least 300 to 350 calories, and snacks should be about 150 to 200. Like the other meals, even snacks should be based on both whole carbohydrates and lean proteins. By eating smaller, yet more frequent, meals with correct proportions of proteins, fats, and carbohydrates, you can manipulate your hormones in favor of obtaining the well-being you want. You'll read more about that below.

The closer one small meal is to the next, the less your glucose levels will nosedive or soar, which means a steady hormone flow on a regular basis. I design my hormone balancing plans with meals timed at every two and a half to three hours, never going more than four waking hours without a balanced meal or "power" snack. Don't be caught without a supply of food to best meet the never-ceasing demands on you.

In addition to stabilizing blood sugars and serotonin production, mini-meals serve your hormones well in another way. Spreading small calorie loads throughout the course of a day appears to trigger your growth hormone, which helps keep your body's metabolism effectively burning calories, building muscle, and metabolizing energy efficiently. When you eat frequent, small meals, your body has a chance to burn those calories for energy instead of storing them as fat—which, in midlife, tends to be of the abdominal variety.

Balancing Power Snack Recipes

Nut Butter Danish	299
Simply Edamame	307
Seeded Tortilla Triangles	308
Roasted Red Pepper Dip	308
Lowfat Hummus	309
Fresh Fruit Tofutti Shake	309

Eat balanced meals and snacks. Eating evenly through the day is not the only important factor in keeping your body working well. Quite obviously, what you eat is also a key. All of the power snacks you see in the accompanying sidebar are designed with a balance of both carbohydrates and proteins—a balance that is vital to your utilizing nutrients optimally for blood sugar stabilization and defusing stress. Forget diets that tell you not to eat one or the other; imbalanced eating only feeds hormonal imbalance.

Earlier, I described a day in the life of Debbie and her erratic, sporadic eating patterns. In addition, she was a twenty-five-year veteran dieter, so she was also confused about what was right nutritionally speaking. She knew how to diet, but not how to "keep it off," and definitely not how to eat in a healthy and energizing way. But once she learned the power that came through eating small, balanced mini-meals through the day—and felt the resulting boost in her metabolism, energy, and moods—she became a believer.

Great Power-Snack Ideas

- Whole grain crackers or whole wheat bread and low-fat cheese (like string cheese, part-skim mozzarella, or Laughing Cow Lite Cheese Wedges)
- Fresh fruit or small box of raisins and low-fat cheese
- Half of a lean turkey or chicken sandwich on whole grain bread
- Plain, nonfat yogurt blended with fruit or all fruit jam, or Stonyfield Farms yogurt
- Whole grain cereal with skim or soy milk
- Wasa bread or Ry-Krisp with light cream cheese and all fruit jam
- Baked low-fat tortilla chips with fat-free bean dip and salsa
- Health Valley graham crackers or whole wheat bread with natural peanut butter
- Popcorn sprinkled with Parmesan cheese
- Homemade low-fat bran muffin with low-fat or skim milk
- Whole grain bread or whole wheat tortilla with sliced turkey and Dijon mustard
- Small pop-top can of water-packed tuna or chicken with whole grain crackers
- Half of a small, whole wheat bagel or English muffin with 2 tbs. light cream cheese
- Fruit shake: skim or soy milk blended with frozen fruit and vanilla
- Trail mix: 1 cup each unsalted dry roasted peanuts and soy nuts, 2 cups unsalted dry roasted shelled pumpkin or sunflower seeds, and 4 cups raisins. (Make it in abundance and bag up into portions of one-fourth of a cup for a whole snack.)

Generally speaking, all the foods you eat supply energy, whether from carbohydrates, proteins, or fats. However, each source provides unique contributions to bodily function and health. Every meal (and power snack) should include both whole food carbohydrates (fresh fruits, vegetables, and whole grains) and lean proteins (meat, fish and seafood, low-fat dairy products, and legumes).

Carbohydrates are 100 percent pure energy—your body's fuel—and the foods that contain them are vital for the production of certain neurotransmitters, particularly vital serotonin. In addition, the fiber that is found in many unprocessed high-carbohydrate foods also helps to regulate bowel function and protects against heart disease and certain types of cancer (you'll read more about whole grains and fiber in chapter 25). In the Hormone Balancing Plan, whole food carbohydrates make up about 55 to 60 percent of your total daily calories.

Protein (including meat, fish, and soybean products) may also be used for energy. However, the body uses protein in more vital ways—to help your brain function and body heal. Protein is a key component of enzymes and hormones. When there are enough calories from other sources, the body uses protein for these functions as well as builds new cells, keeps body fluids in balance, heals and fights infections, and makes skin, hair, and nails more beautiful. If there is a lack of carbohydrate energy, protein's more vital roles are sacrificed, and it's used merely as fuel. About 20 percent of the Hormone Balancing Plan's daily calories are provided by protein.

Protein is made up of amino acids, which are the building blocks for thousands of cell functions. Your body needs twenty different amino acids to function optimally. Some of these are produced

Balancing Lunch Recipes

Terrific Tuna Grill	300
Hot Carrot-Cheese Melt	301
Swiss Stuffed Potatoes	301
Tempeh Sandwiches	302
Tofu Burritos	303
Grilled Turkey and Cheese Sandwich	304
Garden Gazpacho with Salad	304
Chicken of the Sea Sandwich	305
Eggless Salad Sandwich	305
Grilled Tofu Salad	306

in the body; others must be provided by the food that you eat and are thereby essential. Any type of protein will raise the amount of amino acids in your bloodstream, but in order for the amino acids to get into your cells and do their job, you must eat complete proteins that contain all the essential amino acids. Complete proteins are those from animal sources (dairy, meat, and seafood); vegetarian meals and snacks may be made complete by combining plant proteins that complement each other. The body has no storage site for essential amino acids, which is why protein needs to be eaten frequently to supply the body with the tools for all-day building and repair.

Top Ten Protein-Rich Foods

1. Salmon or tuna
2. Egg whites
3. Clams and mussels
4. Chicken or turkey breast
5. Pork tenderloin
6. Cottage, ricotta, or low-fat cheese
7. Lean beef
8. Soy nuts, tempeh, or tofu with grains
9. Lentils (or other beans) with rice
10. Skim or soy milk, yogurt

All protein is not the same. The more amino acids a protein contains, the higher its quality and the better your body can utilize it for producing hormone-balancing neurotransmitters.

CARBOHYDRATES WITH A DIFFERENCE

All carbohydrate isn't the same either. Some carbohydrates are digested and released as energy into the bloodstream slowly and evenly, while others are digested and released quickly — almost too quickly — sending the blood chemistries into gymnastics, triggering a surge of insulin, and preventing the brain from getting the optimum flow of glucose. The best carbohydrates for hormone balance are those that are closest to their unrefined source — fresh vegetables and fruits and whole grains — allowing a better regulation of the blood sugars and brain chemicals. You'll find a listing of these "friendly" carbohydrates on page 223.

An eating plan high in whole-food forms of carbohydrates balanced with low-fat proteins is your best bet for living long and well. Eating the right proteins increases your level of *glucagon*, another hormone that works to prevent insulin surges. If you eat lunches that are high in refined carbohydrates but low in protein, you will throw off the glucagon-insulin balance and may find yourself feeling tired and craving sweets in the afternoon. So keep your metabolism, fat-burning capacity, hormone effectiveness, energy, and concentration *up* (and appetite and cravings *down!*) throughout your day by eating small amounts more often and choosing *whole* carbohydrates balanced with low-fat proteins.

Eat whole food over supplements. You can get your entire daily requirement of vitamin C by just popping a pill. It's easy and convenient. Or you can get the same amount by eating an orange.

So which is better? In most cases, the orange—a "whole food." That's because whole foods—that is, fruits, vegetables, grains, lean meats, and dairy products—have many benefits you simply cannot find in a bottle. While vitamin and nutritional supplements are beneficial in many situations, there are many reasons to favor whole foods as your primary source of nutrition.

Your body needs many nutrients to stay healthy. These include the macronutrients (the protein, carbohydrates, and fats you've just read about) for energy and building and repair of the body, as well as micronutrients (vitamins and minerals) that serve many functions, including disease prevention. Even when taking a daily multivitamin and mineral supplement, you still need to eat a balanced diet with whole foods as the centerpiece. Whole foods are, obviously, the most excellent source of these. They are a complex package that provides many essential nutrients, not just the few you may choose to take in supplement form.

With whole foods, the whole is truly greater than the sum of the parts. Whole foods provide an ideal "mix" of

Balancing Dinner Recipes

Seared Shrimp with Edamame, Corn, and Tomato Saute	310
Marinated Tempeh with Broccoli and Red Peppers	311
Chili Con Tofu	312
Herb Crusted Grouper, Brown Rice Pilaf, and Tuscan Broccoli	313–14
Stir-fried Tofu with Asparagus and Shitakes	315
Chicken Pad Thai	316
BBQ Grilled Tempeh Sandwiches with Chopped Tomato Salad	317
Salmon with Black Bean, Edamame, and Corn Salsa	319
Snapper with Tomato and Feta Cheese with Herb-Roasted Potatoes	320
Spaghetti Pie	321

nutrients, fiber, and other food substances. It's likely that all these work in combination to provide a united health benefit.

For example, an orange provides not only vitamin C but also carotene, folic acid, bioflavonoids, calcium, and simple carbohydrate for energy. A vitamin C supplement is lacking in these other nutrients. Similarly, a glass of milk provides you with protein, calcium, vitamin D, phosphorous, and magnesium. If you take only calcium supplements and skip calcium-rich foods such as dairy products, you miss out on the full complement of nutrients that build healthy bones and so much more.

DO I NEED A MULTIVITAMIN-MINERAL SUPPLEMENT AT ALL?

With that said, we are all able to obtain all the essential nutrients from our daily diets. However, the majority of American women's diets fall considerably short of the basic requirements for total well-being during the menopausal transition. Skipping meals, fast foods, and snacks, as well as chronic dieting and stress, all result in a depletion of the body's stores of vitamins and minerals. So, while you are working on the Hormone Balancing Plan week by week, building a positive way of eating, supplemental capsules may provide a good base. I recommend a basic multivitamin-mineral supplement that contains no more than 150 percent of the daily value for nutrients and certain other single nutrients based on your unique need.

A few examples of vitamin-mineral supplements that supply appropriate dosages are One-a-Day, Theragram, or Centrum. There is no need to spend lots of money on designer vitamins, which are often overloaded with high megadoses that you don't need; in fact, they might hurt you. Too much vitamin A, for example, can damage the eyes and skin and actually promote hip fractures. Megadoses of vitamin D can cause excess calcium in the bloodstream, and too much iron can interfere with immune function and cause liver damage.

Use the meal plan that follows to learn how to fuel your body with the right foods at the right time. The emphasis is not just on what to eat but on how, when, and how much. Focus on eating great foods, prepared in great ways, to work with your body chemistry to bring hormones into balance.

HORMONAL BALANCE PLANNING GUIDE

The Hormone Balancing Meal Plan in this section is your detailed strategy for fueling your body with the right foods at the right time. As you have read, the emphasis is not just on what to eat, but how, when, and how much.

The Hormone Balancing Meal Plan provides approximately 1,500 calories a day. Portion sizes in the plan may need to be adjusted for individual caloric needs. Remember, the number of calories you need depends on your age, size, weight, level of activity, and even stress levels. So don't get caught up in counting every calorie you eat. Instead, focus on eating great foods, prepared in great ways, to propel your body into hormone balance.

You'll be eating plenty of food at meals, plus two or three snacks, properly balanced in whole food, simple and complex carbohydrates, proteins, and fats. But if you get really hungry at other times of the day, have a piece of fruit with one ounce of low-fat or soy cheese or a half cup skim or soy milk. Drink as much water and seltzer as you like, but definitely get in sixty-four ounces every day. Attempt to limit your intake of caffeinated beverages such as coffee, tea, or soda.

My Recommended Supplements for Women in Midlife

Multivitamin and mineral supplement: They should contain at least 100 percent but no more than 150 percent of the established value of vitamins and minerals.

Vitamin E: 200 IU, up to 800 IU (if experiencing hot flashes or breast tenderness, and you have no known history of heart disease)

Vitamin D: 200 IU (if not getting regular sun exposure and if not included in multivitamin or calcium supplement)

Calcium: 1,000 mg (if taking in less than 2 servings of calcium-rich foods a day; calcium citrate is the most absorbable form)

Magnesium: 350 mg (if help is needed to stabilize blood sugars and moods and relieve muscle contractions and cramps)

Vitamin B complex: providing 50 mg of B6 (if help is needed to reduce fatigue, irritability, and emotional stress)

It will take two to three days for your body to stabilize and for you to feel an increase in energy and a regulation of your appetite. In about ten to twelve days, you will notice your body reminding you that it's time for your power snack or meal—about every 2½ to 3 hours. This is a good thing—a sign that your body chemistries are stabilizing.

As you familiarize yourself with the meal plan below, refer to the lists of friendly carbohydrates (page 223), protein-rich foods (page 167), and power snacks (page 165) to refresh your memory of what your best choices are.

Hormone Balancing Meal Plan

Breakfast (within a half hour of arising)

Begin your meal with: 1 serving fresh fruit

Whole carbohydrate: 2 slices whole wheat toast, *or* 1 whole grain English muffin/bagel (may top with 1 tsp. all fruit jam, melted cheese, or lite cream cheese, or use the optional 1 tsp. butter), *or* 2 homemade whole grain low-fat muffins, *or* 1½ cups whole grain cereal with added bran/flaxseed

Protein: 2 ounces part skim or soy cheese, *or* ½ cup low-fat cottage/ricotta cheese, *or* 2 tbs. light cream cheese, *or* 2 eggs (three times/wk), *or* 2 egg whites or egg substitute, *or* 1 cup skim milk for cereal *or* non-fat yogurt

Optional fat: 1 tsp. butter for toast or muffin, *or* 1 tsp. olive or canola oil for cooking, *or* 1 tbs. chopped nuts, *or* 2 tbs. ground flaxseed as topping for cereal or yogurt

Morning snack (2½ to 3 hours after breakfast)

As a whole snack, ¼ cup Trail Mix (page 165), *or* choose a combination of:

Whole carbohydrate: 1 piece of fresh fruit

Protein: 2 oz. part skim or soy cheese, *or* 1 cup non-fat yogurt, *or* 8 ounces skim or soy milk, *or* ½ cup low-fat cottage/ricotta cheese

Lunch (2½ to 3 hours after morning snack)

Begin your meal with 1 piece of fruit, *or* 1 cup cooked vegetables, *or* 1 cup low-fat vegetable soup or vegetable juice

Whole carbohydrate: 2 slices whole grain bread, *or* 1 baked sweet potato, *or* 1 whole wheat pita, *or* 1 whole wheat tortilla, *or* 1 cup brown rice/whole grain pasta

Protein: 3 ounces cooked poultry, fish, seafood, lean beef, tofu or low-fat cheese, *or* ¾ cup cooked legumes

Healthy munchies: Raw vegetables as desired (up to 2 cups) with lemon juice, vinegar, mustard, salsa, or no-oil salad dressing

Optional fat: May use 1 tbs. salad dressing, *or* 1 tsp. olive or canola oil making your own salad dressing or to cook with, *or* you may use 1 tsp. butter for bread or potato, *or* 2 tbs. sour cream on potato, *or* 1 tbs. chopped nuts or 2 tbs. ground flaxseed sprinkled on foods

Afternoon snack (2½ to 3 hours after lunch)

Whole carbohydrate: 1 piece of fruit, *or* 5 whole-grain crackers, *or* ½ whole wheat pita, *or* 1 ounce baked tortilla chips (with salsa, if desired), *or* 1 slice whole wheat bread

Protein: 1 ounce part-skim or soy cheese (on bread), *or* 1 ounce lean meat, *or* ⅓ cup low-fat bean dip (with chips above), *or* ½ cup non-fat yogurt, *or* ¼ cup low-fat cottage/ricotta cheese

Healthy munchies: raw veggies (up to one cup)

Dinner (2½ to 3 hours after afternoon snack)

Begin with 1 piece of fruit or ½ cup mixed fruit, *or* 1 cup low-fat vegetable soup *and* then enjoy another serving of fruit, *or* 1 cup non-starchy vegetables with dinner

Whole carbohydrate: ½ cup cooked brown rice or whole-grain pasta, *or* ½ cup starchy vegetables, *or* 1 small baked sweet potato

Protein: 2–3 ounces cooked skinless poultry, seafood, fish, lean beef, or tofu, *or* ½ cup cooked legumes

Healthy munchies: Raw vegetables (up to 2 cups) as desired with lemon juice, vinegar, salsa, or no-oil salad dressing

Optional fat: May use 1 tbs. salad dressing, *or* 1 tsp. olive or canola oil making your own salad dressing or to cook with, *or* you may use 1 tsp. butter for bread or potato, *or* 2 tbs. sour cream on potato, *or* 1 tbs. chopped nuts or 2 tbs. ground flaxseed sprinkled on foods

Night snack (at least ½ hour before bedtime)

Whole carbohydrate: ¾ cup whole grain cereal, *or* 1 slice whole grain bread

Protein: ½ cup skim or soy milk or non-fat yogurt (with cereal), *or* 1 ounce lean meat, *or* 1 ounce low-fat or soy cheese (melted atop bread)

Putting Your Plan to Work

Now let's put that plan to work. Below is a sample menu for one day, following the guidelines above.

7:00 A.M.

Breakfast of 2 slices whole grain toast topped with 2 ounces of melted, low-fat cheese, and 1 peach

9:30 to 10:00 A.M.

¼ cup trail mix

12:00 noon to 12:30 P.M.

Lunch of 1 sliced orange as an appetizer, 1 turkey tortilla roll (2 ounces of turkey and 1 ounce of cheese rolled into 1 whole wheat, fat-free tortilla, spread with Dijon mustard, with shredded romaine lettuce and tomato), plus cut-up raw broccoli, carrots, and red peppers to munch on.

3:00 P.M.

Power shake made with ½ cup frozen berries blended with ½ cup yogurt, a dash of vanilla and 1 tbs. ground flaxseed.

6:00 P.M.

Appetizer of 8-ounce glass of V–8 juice, then 3 ounces grilled fish or chicken, ½ cup steamed brown rice, 1 cup cooked asparagus, a baby spinach and tomato salad drizzled with low-fat balsamic dressing, ½ cup blueberries for dessert

Half hour before bed

½ cup whole grain cereal topped with 1 tbs. ground flaxseed and ½ cup skim or soy milk

HORMONE BALANCING
ACTION STEPS—WEEK THREE

✔ *Evaluate last week's diary.* Compare that diary to the "Hormone Balancing Eat Right Prescription" you've just read and note adjustments you might want to make in your timing and/or balance of meals and snacks. After you've evaluated your present eating habits and have found your weak spots, you can get on your way toward eating strategically. Start a new diary this week.

✔ *Eat early.* Choose to eat a balanced breakfast every day— within the first half hour of arising. Choose one of the breakfasts on pages 163 or 171 or creatively put together your own, being sure to have both a whole carbohydrate and a low-fat protein each time.

✔ *Eat often.* Have a power meal or power snack every 2½ to 3 hours. Choose one of the power snack ideas on page 165 or put together your own. Record them in your diary for this week, adding any comments about feelings or symptoms.

✔ *Eat balanced.* In addition to a balanced breakfast, be sure that *every* meal and snack provides a balance of whole carbohydrates and lean proteins—*every time!* Ask yourself "Where's my protein?" If it's just a salad, it's not enough. If it's just a piece of fruit, even for a snack, you need more. If it's just a piece of chicken, you need some carbohydrate.

✔ *Eat whole foods.* Stop for a moment and acknowledge food as your divine source of nutrition. Okay. Now refer to the supplement guide on page 170 to determine which supplements, if any, are necessary to uniquely fit your needs. Pick them up at the market or pharmacy and get started with the right supplements to help nourish you while upgrading your eating with the Hormone Balancing Plan.

✔ *Body-spirit balance step.* While feeding your physical body in new nourishing ways, consider optimal food for your spirit.

In your time of quiet—in the morning, in the evening, or during a break in your day—reflect on a verse from Scripture, a prayer, an inspirational reading, the words of a hymn, or the like. One place you may begin is with this Scripture:

> *The eyes of all look to you,*
> > *and you give them their food at the proper time.*
> *You open your hand*
> > *and satisfy the desires of every living thing.*
> > > Psalm 145:15–16

Mom Was Right: Eat Your Fruits and Vegetables

Fruits and vegetables come closer than any other category of food to behaving like a fountain of youth. I cannot emphasize enough the importance for women in midlife to increase their consumption of these beauties and their need to choose broadly from among the richly colored options.

In addition to vitamins and minerals, fresh fruits and vegetables contain hundreds to thousands of plant compounds called *phytonutrients* (nutrients in plants) or *phytochemicals*, all of which are vital to getting us well and keeping us well. Although still somewhat of a mystery, these food chemicals work to power our immune systems to keep us vital, lovely, and protected against diseases such as cancer, heart disease, osteoporosis, and diabetes, as well as stabilizing and boosting our hormone production.

Wondrously, these phytonutrients are packed into everyday foods we eat—or should eat. It is estimated that there are over nine thousand health-promoting plant-based substances, but at the moment only a few more than a hundred phytonutrients have been identified. You'll be reading a lot about these power substances in the coming pages—nutrients such as bioflavonoids, beta-carotene, phenols, lycopene, indoles, proanthocyanidins, and phytoestrogens—nature's pharmacy of hormones.

COLOR ME HEALTHY

While many of these phytonutrients are already cropping up in supplements, research continues to show that food, particularly fruits and vegetables, is still their best source. In fact, studies have often shown that phytonutrient supplements have little benefit, as a team of scientists reported in the December 2001 issue of *Journal of the American Dietetic Association*. Instead, one of the best guarantees to good health is to shop the supermarket with your eye on color.

These days, it's a beautiful and tempting sight to behold the expansive array of colorful produce in the supermarket aisles. Although the brighter the better for their phyto-protection, even the paler members of this community — garlic, onions, leeks, cabbage, celery, and the like — have many notable health-promoting virtues.

TEN-A-DAY KEEPS THE DOCTOR AWAY

No doubt you have encountered the government's "five-a-day" campaign. At most, only a third of the population meets that healthy goal. Yet, based on the research findings that are coming in, I am encouraging you to *double* that. If you check the Food Pyramid, you will see that five servings a day of fruits and vegetables is the bare minimum recommended for achieving a wholesome diet. As far as I am concerned, *ten* servings or more is optimal for hormonal health maintenance.

Getting in ten servings a day of produce is not too difficult, once you realize what a serving is: one medium apple, banana, or orange, half a grapefruit, a quarter of a cantaloupe, a cup of raw, leafy vegetables, half a cup of cooked or chopped raw vegetables or fruit, and six ounces of fruit or vegetable juice. But merely counting servings of fruits and vegetables, although a good start, is not enough. The key is eating an ample and colorful variety to be sure you are eating enough of the different phytochemicals needed to stimulate hormone production and the metabolic pathways of genes in the different organs where fruits and vegetables have their beneficial effects.

Here is a sample day to give you an idea of how ten servings can happen:

(1) Start your day with a small glass of juice, right after your water.
(2) Add fruit to your breakfast cereal, yogurt, power shake, or French toast.
(3) and (4)–Snack on cheese, yogurt, or lean meat with whole fruit, fruit salad, or vegetables like baby carrots for both a morning and afternoon snack.
(5) and (6)–Have a big salad with lunch or dinner (that will count for at least two!).
(7) Drink a vegetable juice (like V–8, carrot, or tomato) or fruit juice, or have a piece of fruit as an appetizer before your lunch and dinner meals.
(8) and (9)–Dine on main courses that include stir-fried, stewed, grilled, or steamed vegetables (just a cup will give another two!).
(10) Have fruit—like berries, peaches, or mangoes—as your dessert!

UNIQUELY POWERFUL

Not all members of the fruit and vegetable group are alike. Virtually all contain antioxidants, but each one has unique properties that provide combinations of substances with unique effects on human biology. (For a list of the most potent, see below.) It's not difficult to take in high doses of antioxidants in modest portions of fruits and vegetables. The color of the pulp or skin is a sign of the type of phyto-protection within. Generally, highest in antioxidants are those with the most vivid colors, such as berries and green leafy vegetables.

Every day, try for at least one serving from these different color groups:

• **Orange**, including carrots, mangoes, cantaloupe, pumpkin, winter squash, and sweet potatoes, rich in the cancer-fighter *alpha-carotene*, along with *beta-carotene*, which protect the skin against free-radical damage and promotes repair of damaged DNA.

- **Orange/yellow,** including oranges, peaches, papaya, and nectarines, which provide *beta-cryptothanxin*, which supports intracellular communication and helps prevent heart disease.

- **Yellow/green,** including spinach, collards, romaine lettuce, corn, green peas, avocado, and honeydew, which are sources of the carotenoids *lutein* and *zeaxanthin*. These are strongly linked to a reduced risk of cataracts and age-related macular degeneration, the leading cause of preventable blindness in developed countries.

- **Deep green,** including broccoli, brussels sprouts, cabbage, kale, and bok choy. These are rich in cancer-blocking chemicals like *sulforaphane, isocyanate,* and *indoles,* which inhibit the action of carcinogens—specifically those involved in breast cancer.

- **White/green,** including garlic, shallots, onions, leeks, celery, asparagus, pears, green apples, and green grapes. The onion family contains *allicin,* which has antitumor and blood-pressure lowering properties. Other foods in this group contain antioxidant flavonoids like *quercetin* and *kaempferol.* White wine is in this category.

- **Red,** including tomatoes (especially cooked tomato products), pink grapefruit, and watermelon, which are rich in the carotenoid *lycopene,* a potent scavenger of gene-damaging free radicals that helps cut the risk of several types of cancer as well as protect against heart and lung disease. The latest evidence suggests that cooking boosts lycopene levels, so that pasta with red sauce is an excellent source.

- **Red/purple,** including red and blue grapes, blueberries, strawberries, beets, eggplant, red cabbage, red peppers, plums, and red apples, which are loaded with powerful antioxidants called *anthocyanins.* They have been shown to delay cellular aging and help the heart by blocking the formation of blood clots; they also help to control blood pressure. Red wine fits in this category.

The trick is to include as many plant-based colors in your daily diet as possible. In many cases, that means eating the colorful skins, the richest sources of protective phytonutrients, along with the paler flesh. Thus, try to avoid peeling foods like apples, red pears, and eggplant lest you lose their most concentrated source of beneficial chemicals. Wash them well instead under cold running water. (I do recommend peeling if the skins have been waxed.)

Heat does not destroy large amounts of the healthy phytochemicals as it does some vitamins. In some cases, as in tomatoes' lycopene or carrots' beta-carotene, cooking actually concentrates the nutrients and makes them more available to the body.

TIPS TO RETAIN NUTRIENTS

- Buy vegetables that are as fresh as possible — in season and locally grown whenever you can.
- When fresh isn't available, frozen is the next best choice. Avoid those frozen with butter or sauces.
- Use well-washed peelings and outer leaves of vegetables whenever possible because of the high concentration of nutrients found within them.

Colorful Vegetable Recipes

Orange:
Terrific Tuna Grill	300
Hot Carrot-Cheese Melt	301
Miso-Carrot Dressing	307

Orange/yellow:
Fresh Fruit Tofutti Shake (with Peaches)	309

Yellow/green:
Edamame, Corn and Tomato Saute	310
Black Bean and Corn Salsa	318

Deep Green:
Grilled Tofu Salad	306
Edamame, Corn, and Tomato Saute	310
Marinated Tempeh with Broccoli and Red Peppers	311
Tuscan Broccoli	314
Garlic Spinach	317
Chicken Pad Thai	316

White/green:
Stir-Fried Tofu with Asparagus and Shiitakes	315

Red:
Garden Gazpacho	304
Chili Con Tofu	312
Chopped Tomato Salad	318

Red/purple:
Breakfast Shake with Berries	296

- Store vegetables in airtight containers in the refrigerator.
- Do not store vegetables in water; too many vitamins are lost.
- Cook vegetables on the highest heat possible, in the least amount of water possible, and for the shortest time possible. Steaming, microwaving, and stir-frying are the best cooking methods; crockpot cooking is the worst.
- Cook vegetables until tender crisp, not mushy. Overcooked vegetables lose their flavor along with their nutrients.

WHAT ABOUT PHYTOCHEMICAL SUPPLEMENTS?

It is alluring to just take herbal or food supplements that promise to contain beneficial phytonutrients, believing that because they are "natural," they are also naturally safe. In theory, plant-derived chemicals are less potent than drugs and so seem safer. But in reality, isolated plant chemicals in supplement form are often taken in much greater volume, so they actually have drug-like dangers.

While people have always been safely eating foods, there is no history of people consuming isolated and concentrated components from plants in large amounts on a daily basis. There are no long-term studies that indicate this is safe to do, particularly for women who have, or who are at risk for, diseases such as breast cancer.

Let's take the example of broccoli. This dark green vegetable contains the phytochemical *isothiocyanates*. In laboratory studies, these have been shown to retard cancer cell growth. Studies also indicate that people who eat broccoli and related vegetables may have a lower risk of colon cancer. Broccoli mimics the breast cancer-preventive drug *tamoxifen*—serving as an estrogen receptor blocker—and contains substances that make estrogen less potent and that serve as a "protective shield" of sorts for the cell.

Super Antioxidant Fruits and Vegetables

Blueberries	Strawberries
Blackberries	Spinach
Garlic	Raspberries
Kale	Dried plums (formerly known as prunes!)
Pomegranate	
Cranberries	Raisins

However, it's too early to tell for sure what substances (isothiocyanate or some other component) may be responsible for the apparent benefit. Moreover, it is not known if taking such an ingredient by itself, as in a supplement, will result in the same benefits as is apparent in those who eat the actual food. Remember, generally the whole food is the best and most nutrient-filled choice.

So a word of caution is called for: *Avoid nutritional supplements and powders that claim to have the same active ingredients as foods.* At best, they may not help you; at worst, these products may contain unknown chemicals that could be harmful. In fact, some of the food components themselves may actually be detrimental to your health when taken as an isolated substance. For example, some studies found an increased risk of lung cancer in smokers who took beta-carotene supplements. Meanwhile, people who consumed adequate amounts of fruits and vegetables (which contain beta-carotene in a mix with many other nutrients) were found to have a lower incidence of cancer.

There's much data to suggest that a diet high in fruits and vegetables will reduce your risk of cancer, heart disease, stroke, and many other diseases. But there is little evidence to suggest the degree of protection individual phytochemical supplements may offer. Until more is known about these, you are better off eating whole foods rather than supplements of these substances. This is especially true with the powerful phytoestrogens — a little is great, a lot is not necessarily better.

HORMONE BALANCING
ACTION STEPS: WEEK FOUR

Eat more fruits and vegetables for their anti-inflammatory phytochemicals and brain-boosting vitamins and minerals.

✔ *Continue to choose foods and portions for your meals and snacks based on the principles of eating early, eating often, and eating balanced.* Record what you eat and any exercise you may do; record also how you are feeling in your Food-Feelings-and-Findings Journal. When you experience a negative symptom, evaluate your food diary for a pattern. When you notice feeling especially good, look for a pattern in your choices preceding it.

✔ *Each day, strive to achieve the goal of eating ten servings of fruits and vegetables.* Use the meal planning guide in chapter 19 to help give you ideas.

✔ *Each day, check off the vegetables and fruits from the "family of color" to which they belong.* Determine which colors need more of your attention and add foods of these colors to your grocery list for next week, based on what might be in season. If you are looking for a place to start, begin by eating some fresh broccoli this week. Try the recipe on page 314 for a starter.

✔ *Look at your sleep patterns.* If you aren't getting at least seven to eight hours of sleep each night, try to get to bed by 9:00 P.M. at least one night this week. Going to bed early is the *best* way to catch up on sleep!

✔ *Body-spirit balance step.* Connect with an encouraging friend this week and share the three top changes you have made and how you are feeling as a result. Consult the "fuel gauge" once again (on page 141) and compare how you are doing now to when you first began the Hormone Balancing Plan. You may want to reflect on this Scripture, thanking God for meeting the desires of your heart and for renewing your strength as you come into hormonal balance:

> Praise the Lord, O my soul,
>   and forget not his benefits . . .
> who satisfies your desires with good things
>   so that your youth is renewed like the eagle's.
>   Psalm 103:2–5

TURN DOWN THE THERMOSTAT WITH PHYTOESTROGENS

Becky's husband was the impetus behind our beginning to counsel together to develop a midlife nutritional strategy for her fifty-year-old body, saying that it was going to be a much better investment than paying the exorbitant air-conditioning bills. She explained her main issue, hot flashes, by telling me about missing blowing out the fifty candles on her birthday cake (really, fifty candles!) because she was in the ladies room stripping off dripping clothes. She was logging in eight to ten serious flashes a day — with no end in sight — and it was interfering with just about everything in her life.

Hormone Replacement Therapy was not an option for Becky, and she had tried just about every herbal remedy known to man, with no relief. Her plea: Was there anything nutritionally she could do?

By maintaining a healthy diet of foods rich in phytoestrogens (plant hormones), we can mirror what women in traditional cultures such as India and Japan have been doing for centuries. Like them, we can hope to enjoy strong bones, healthy hearts, and minimal to no menopausal symptoms. Over four thousand media articles were released last year alone showing the health impact of these powerful substances.

A phytoestrogen is a type of plant chemical we just read about — one with "hormone-like" action. Its activity is relatively weak compared with that of estrogen taken as a medication;

prescription estrogen is more than a hundred times stronger than phytoestrogens. Yet, the phytoestrogens work in an amazing way with a double balancing impact: If estrogen levels are low, they exert an estrogenic effect; if estrogen levels are high, phytoestrogens appear to occupy estrogen receptor sites in the body, "fooling" it into believing it has enough, thus preventing further production.

This estrogen-blocking side is just one of the reasons why they are so beneficial for perimenopause—a time when estrogen levels are as apt to be as high (dominant) as they are low. In addition, the phytoestrogens may serve as a sound defensive strategy against foreign estrogens, such as those coming from hormones added to animal feed and pesticides. They may be able to occupy estrogen receptors, blocking access to these stronger *xenoestrogens*.

Almost all fruits, vegetables, and cereal grains contain phytoestrogens of varying strengths and makeup. One type, the isoflavones, are most beneficial to hormone balance. Isoflavones (genestein, daidzein, biochanin A, and formononetin) are found in legumes such as lentils, chickpeas, and most noticeably, soybeans. Bacteria in the gut convert isoflavones into substances that have an estrogenic action, although they are not themselves hormones.

High Phytoestrogen Foods

- Soy and other legumes, such as chickpeas, lentils, azuki beans, kidney beans, and peas
- Garlic
- Seeds, including flaxseed, sesame, pumpkin, poppy, caraway, and sunflower
- Grains, like wheat, rice, oats, barley, and rye
- Fruits, including citrus fruits, cherries, plums, berries, pomegranates, and apples
- Vegetables, including celery, broccoli, green beans, carrots, rhubarb, and potatoes
- Sprouts like alfalfa and mung bean sprouts
- Certain herbs and spices, such as cinnamon, sage, red clover, anise, fennel, and parsley

Because soybeans are especially rich in phytoestrogens (containing the genestein and daidzein types), they have been studied extensively. An average Japanese woman's daily intake of isoflavones is between 20 and 80 mg a day, Asian women overall take in about 45 mg per day, while American women generally consume only 1–3 mg per day. That's a huge difference! Researchers at the Northern California Cancer Center have found that few American women eat sufficient soy foods to get enough isoflavones to positively affect their health.

Other phytoestrogens include *lignans*, most noticeably in oilseeds, especially flax (which is another reason why flaxseed is such a nutritional powerhouse), and *coumestans*, found primarily in alfalfa and mung bean sprouts.

SOY STORY

With all the media attention around soy, you would think we would eat more soy foods than we do. But the problem is that it is unfamiliar to many of us; most Americans did not grow up with soy foods on the family table. Only recently have tasty soy products been showing up in the neighborhood grocery stores, so it's taken extra work, determination, and a good deal of courage to even find or try them.

Let's face it, soy has a pretty grim reputation. Its most enduring image in this country is that of a '60s health food, with its heavy, bland lentil-bulgur stews, noodle loaves, and tofu casseroles. Tofu still represents the worst of the era to many people, which might explain why only 2 percent of the two billion bushels of soybeans grown in the United States is consumed as human food, with half of that going abroad. The rest ends up in livestock feed and other nonfood products.

If you are unfamiliar with (or turned off by!) soy, try some of the recipes on pages 296–321, which showcase delicious ways to use soy. (Many recipes are based in Asian cuisine.) Certainly billions of Asians have found much to love about soy. In China the word for soybean is *dadou*, which means "greater bean."

SOY PRIMER

Soy is unique among plant foods in that it supplies all the essential amino acids. It also provides protein without the high levels of saturated fats in red meats. Soy has two things you need to care about: soy protein and isoflavones. Although it's still unclear exactly how isoflavones and other soy compounds work to protect against disease and to balance hormones, an ever-growing body of research makes a strong case for their benefits.

Isoflavone concentrations vary from food to food. The highest are in whole-bean products that haven't been highly processed. The more processing done to soy, the fewer phytoestrogens remain in the food, as is the case with many of the textured vegetable proteins or meat look-alikes you may have had at some point along the way. So, try to choose the foods closest to soy's natural state. Soybeans are by far the best, and edamame (young soybean pods) or tempeh (a fermented mixture of whole soybeans and a grain such as millet, barley, or rice) are next—and great tasting to boot! The next best forms of soy are soy nuts, tofu, miso, soy flour, and some soy milks and cheeses.

There's no way to know a food's precise level of phytoestrogens (unless it's on the label), but if you put your focus onto getting enough soy protein each day (25 g), you'll get plenty of isoflavones too (the goal being about 45 mg per day).

If you are buying a soy food, look for the amount of protein per serving in the "Nutritional Facts" box. If it's a food that is all soy (such as tofu or edamame), all the protein will be soy as well. If there are other ingredients—such as in energy bars or cereals—look specifically for the amount of soy protein per serving. If it's not mentioned or there is no indication as to the actual amount, most likely there's not much.

Edamame beans are served as a starter at many Japanese restaurants and are delicious sources of protein. If you think you don't like soy, give these a try; they taste a lot like baby

More Recipes with Soy

Edamame

Simply Edamame	307
Edamame, Corn, and Tomato Saute	310
Black Bean, Corn, and Edamame Salsa	318

Tempeh

Tempeh Sandwiches	302
BBQ Grilled Tempeh Sandwiches	302
Marinated Tempeh with Broccoli and Red Peppers	311

Tofu

Tofu Burritos	303
Eggless Salad Sandwich	305
Grilled Tofu Salad with Miso-Carrot Dressing	306–7
Roasted Red Pepper Dip	308
Fresh Fruit Tofutti Shake	309
Lowfat Hummus	309
Chili Con Tofu	312–13
Stir-fried Tofu with Asparagus and Shitakes	315
Chicken Pad Thai	316

lima beans. Pods are harvested when they are still young and tender.
The beans, when steamed and salted, are great for snacking. They
are slightly lower in isoflavones than mature beans, but one cup of
the shelled edamame still gives 25 grams of soy protein. Nowadays
you can find them fresh or frozen in many supermarkets as well as
specialty food stores.

To prepare, you simply steam or boil the soybeans in their pods
for about five minutes. Then lightly salt them, and they're ready
to eat. You don't eat the pod; rather, open it up and pick out the
soybeans, or place the whole pod in your mouth and scrape out the
edible beans. You'll be amazed at how good they are! Or you can
use them in stir-fry, soup, a salad, a pasta dish, or a succotash. Find
more recipes for edamame on pages 307, 310, and 318.

Tempeh is chewy but tender. It's almost meat-like and ties with
edamame as my very favorite form of soy to use in cooking. It makes
for a great sandwich (really!) and can be added to stir-fry, soups,
stews, or chili. It is found in the refrigerated or the freezer section of
a natural foods store and comes in both a plain and flavored variety
and in a single or three-grain type. Tempeh gives you 5.5 grams of
protein per ounce. Try the recipes on pages 302 and 311.

Tofu, made from curdled fresh soy milk, is a white and silky
block that can be bought as extra firm, firm, or silken. Firm tofu
is easier to cut into cubes, so is ideal for stir-fry and soup. The soft
silken type is best in dishes that are blended, such as shakes, pud-
dings, and dips, and it is also lower in fat. Tofu provides 2 to 4.5
grams of protein per ounce.

Tofu has no real taste of its own, so its flavor is dependent on
what you cook it with. This makes it wonderfully versatile and definitely worth trying — or trying anew! Experiment with some of the
recipes noted in the recipe index on page 188.

Miso, a dark brown or golden soybean paste, is a combination
of soybeans and a grain (such as rice) that is aged for one to three
years. Because of its strong, rich flavor, miso can be used in small
quantities — a positive because it carries a lot of sodium. It can
be added to stocks or glazes or used as a base for salad dressings
and dips. Mixed with water, it can make a soothing broth on its
own. It is sold in a plastic container at Asian markets as well as

in most supermarkets and provides about 4 grams of protein per ounce—enough for about two cups of soup.

Soy nuts are roasted mature soybeans. You'll find salted and unsalted, dry roasted and those roasted with oil. I prefer those that are unsalted, dry roasted. They're tasty and loaded with isoflavones and soy protein—20 grams per one-third cup—but they need to be eaten with caution as they are also high in calories and higher in fat (albeit not a saturated one) than my usually suggested lean proteins. I make my Trail Mix with soy nuts; you'll find the recipe on page 165. The same red flag applies to soy nut butter, which looks like peanut butter but with a slightly different taste. Although it would never be confused with a peanut butter and jelly (at least by my family!), two tablespoons of soy butter spread on toast makes for a deliciously easy breakfast. Try topping the soy butter toast with sliced banana or all fruit jam.

Soy milk can be used in cooking in the same way as cow's milk; once mixed with other ingredients, it is hard to taste the difference. Soy milk is a creamy liquid made from crushed whole soybeans and is often sold in shelf-stable containers, either plain or sweetened and flavored. Each of the various brands of soy milk tastes different, so don't give up if you don't love the first one you buy. You may enjoy those that are in the refrigerated dairy case more than those shelf-stable brands. An average serving of soy milk (about one cup) has 7 grams of protein. I use it in power shakes and as cooking liquid for my oatmeal.

Soy cheese is made from tofu and comes in great flavors like pepper jack and Swiss. One of my favorite brands is Veggie-Slices.

Soy yogurt (also sold as cultured soy) is made by adding active yogurt cultures to soy

Recipes with Soy

Miso

Grilled Tofu Salad with Miso-Carrot Dressing — 306–7

Soy Nuts

Trail Mix — 165
Nut Butter Danish — 299

Soy Milk

Breakfast Shake — 296
Hot Apple-Cinnamon Oatmeal — 298

Soy Cheese

Toasted Cheese and Pears — 297
Terrific Tuna Grill — 300
Hot Carrot-Cheese Melt — 301
Grilled Turkey and Cheese Sandwich — 304

milk. It has a similar protein content as cow's milk yogurt, about 5 grams per cup.

Soy sauce, the salty dark brown sauce, available in many varieties, combines the liquid of fermented soybeans with wheat. *Tamari* is made with soybeans alone. You do get some protein from these sauces (about 1.5 to 3 grams per two tablespoons), but they're completely devoid of isoflavones. Moreover, the high salt content begs a limit to the quantity you use.

Soy flour is made from ground roasted soybeans and can be used in place of white flour in recipes for baked goods like breads and muffins. Substitute it for a third to a quarter of the amount of regular flour. It's very high in protein, providing 10 to 14 grams per quarter cup.

Don't bother to eat soy ice cream in the name of hormone balance; it has little to no protein and is packed with sugar. Eat it if you like it, period, and still only occasionally. Soy margarine is the same deal—no protein, no isoflavones, and all fat (just like regular margarine) because it's made from soybean oil. (Olive oil is still the very best choice for an added fat.)

HOW MUCH SOY?

Again, as a general guideline, I suggest including 45 mg of isoflavones in your diet each day. You could get this from just a half cup of edamame, two ounces of tempeh, three ounces of tofu, or two cups soy milk; it doesn't require massive amounts. One study showed a 40 percent reduction in hot flashes from this "dose"; another study showed that a higher amount (60 mg) of isoflavones were required to achieve a significant reduction in hot flashes. There was also a study that showed 20 grams of soy protein per day reduce blood pressure and improve lipids, reducing LDL cholesterol and triglycerides and increasing HDL cholesterol. Other studies have shown positive impact on vaginal dryness and irritation—even changes in high FSH levels—with just these small doses.

Isoflavones have also been indicated to be beneficial for preventing the long-term health risks from osteoporosis, heart disease, and diabetes for post-menopausal women. These natural plant estrogens promote growth of new bone tissue and slow bone loss. The isoflavones in soy are identical to a drug called *ipriflavone*, used as a synthetic isoflavone for bone loss, so there's good reason to believe soy's isoflavones can improve bone health. At the end of one study, perimenopausal women who took isoflavones lost significantly less spinal bone than those who took a placebo.

Just as supplemental estrogen appears to protect against the bone loss that leads to osteoporosis, studies have found that soy may do the same, at least for the six-month period measured. If that protection continued for many years, women may have been able to lower their risk of osteoporosis just by eating soy, with no HRT and the risks associated with it.

Regarding other long-term health issues, another recent study found that a nonprescription red clover extract (Promensil) containing 40 mg of isoflavones boosted the elasticity of arterial walls as effectively as HRT. (The loss of arterial elasticity, which often occurs in menopause, raises a woman's risk for heart disease.) And a study released in June 2002 showed that soy could help stabilize blood sugars and insulin levels in women prone to diabetes.

THE DANGERS OF SOY

The many promises for soy have led many women to begin taking soy supplements, something I *don't* advise. We have already discussed the concerns of taking supplements compared to eating whole foods, and it's a dangerous game when it comes to soy. Some women have developed goiter or symptoms of hyperthyroidism while consuming large amounts of soy supplements. If you are taking thyroid hormone to correct hypothyroidism, large amounts of soy may prevent you from absorbing the medication properly; soy or isoflavone supplements more easily allow an overdose. And since isoflavones play the role of estrogen, there is a chance that they could cause a proliferation of breast cells and actually increase the risk of breast cancer in the same way supplemental estrogen can.

Because of this risk, there is a great deal of confusion and controversy surrounding the inclusion of soy in the diets of those women with estrogen-positive, postmenopausal breast cancer—especially those being treated with the drug tamoxifen. Though a few cancer specialists advise women in this category to avoid soy foods because of the weak estrogen compounds they contain, many believe that one or two servings a day of whole soy foods (such as those that the Japanese consume) will not be harmful. I follow the research in this field closely, and I continue to advise eating one or two servings of whole soy foods a day, even for women who have had breast cancer.

Not surprisingly, I do *not* recommend soy powders or soy pills that contain isolated isoflavones, nor do I recommend soy foods with extra isoflavones added to them. I also prefer to stay with the traditional Asian soy foods—edamame, tofu, tempeh, and miso—as compared to the more processed soy protein powders. Again, just because some is good does not mean that *more* is better; it can sometimes be lethal.

If soy has an *anticancer* effect, I believe that it comes from all the beneficial compounds in soy working together—at the levels consumed in Asia. Going with the research implication that taking a daily 40 mg isoflavone supplement may give health benefits and symptom relief, then consuming 40 mg of dietary isoflavones (one serving of tofu or one cup of soy milk supplies 30 mg to 40 mg) would be equally effective but without the risk that comes through taking isolated substances. Until more tests are done, stick to moderate amounts of *whole* soy foods.

Bottom line on soy: I recommend whole soy foods only; avoid supplements. *Definitely* avoid supplements if you have an increased risk of breast cancer.

HORMONE BALANCING
ACTION STEPS: WEEK FIVE

Have a variety of phytoestrogen-rich foods.

✔ *Review your Food-Feeling-and-Findings Journal from last week.* Are there times of the day when you are hungry or crave certain foods? How about your moods and energy? Are there moments when you are particularly high or low? Do you see any routine or food triggers for perimenopausal symptoms such as hot flashes, headaches, or insomnia? Pay particular attention to positive changes toward the end of this phytoestrogen-boosting week.

- *Adjust the timing of your eating to best undergird your blood sugars.* Also review your diary for food choices that may contribute to better stabilization, such as a better balance of whole (and less refined) carbohydrates and lean proteins at every meal and snack.

- *Circle any phytoestrogen-rich foods you may have consumed.* Smiley-face the days that you had at least two servings, and red-star the days you had less than two servings or none.

- *Look at the list of high phytoestrogen foods.* Choose those you could feasibly insert into the deficient days you highlighted above. Choose at least two foods that are new to you and add those to your weekly grocery list. Consult pages 295–321 for recipes to make the process delicious.

- *Increase walking to twenty minutes a day.* You can do this either at one time or in two ten-minute sessions. If you are already exercising aerobically, do the twenty-minute walk at another time.

- *Body-spirit balance step.* Use your walking as a time to reflect on the changes you are making and experiencing. Pay attention to your self-talk—is it negative? We can be our own worst enemy or our own best friend; it's all revealed in how we talk to ourselves. It's amazing how often we put ourselves down throughout the day, and it's time to stop! We need to replace the negative thoughts with positive ones. Next time you catch yourself thinking that there is no hope, that you can never change, or that you cannot follow this hormone balance plan, fight back! Immediately appeal to God to correct your thinking, compliment yourself on what you have accomplished, marvel at how specially you were created, and remember your destination: hormone balance. The following passage from God's Word may give you inspiration this week:

  For I know the plans I have for you . . . plans to give you hope and a future.

  Jeremiah 29:11

GET FIRED UP
WITH WATER!

If you do nothing else in your quest for hormone balance but begin to drink water each day—and drink a lot of it—you will experience a phenomenal boost in your energy and sense of well-being. Few of my clients think of water as their most important health enhancement, yet many of the symptoms of fatigue and fuzzy thinking that we blame on too little estrogen, too little sleep, and too much stress are simply the result of chronic dehydration.

At the end of a long day, when you feel rotten and headachy and unmotivated to exercise—in a strange zone between sore and numb—your body is crying out to be hydrated. Chances are you have only drunk enough water to wash down a few aspirin and have had little else to drink since that coffee or diet soda this morning. You have been breathing dry, air-conditioned, or heated air all day, and the chronic stress in your routine has caused some moments of intense perspiration. And of course, you've been losing fluids through the day through normal body functions—fluids that haven't been replaced. You're parched!

THIRSTING FOR WELLNESS

It may be hard to believe, but the number one factor in fatigue is dehydration. Water is an essential nutrient—one of the big six, numbering right along with carbohydrates, protein, fat, vitamins, and minerals. Without food, a person can survive (although not well!) for days, even months. But without water, the human body can survive only three to five days.

Every cell in your body relies on water to dilute biochemicals, vitamins, and minerals to just the right concentrations and to transport the nutrients throughout your body. Water is the only liquid we consume that doesn't require the body to work to metabolize or excrete it. Even fresh juices don't provide the solid benefits of pure, wonderful water, since they require your body to process the substances they contain.

In addition, water helps you digest food and maintain proper bowel function and waste elimination. Being a mild laxative, water actually activates the fiber you eat, allowing it to form a bulky mass that passes through the gastrointestinal tract easily and quickly. Without proper water, fiber becomes a difficult-to-pass "glue" in your colon! Big water drinkers get less colon and bladder cancer.

And water is good for your heart too. In a recent study, drinking at least five glasses of water per day was shown to reduce the risk of fatal heart attack. Drinking other fluids, such as tea, juice, coffee, or milk, did not have the same protective effect as drinking water. Water helps to thin the blood, making it less likely to clot and cause blockages. In that study, men who drank at least five glasses of water per day had a 54 percent lower risk of dying from a heart attack compared to men who drank only two glasses of water per day. Women who drank five glasses per day had a 41 percent lower risk of heart attack death.

In addition, because water is also vital for maintaining proper muscle tone, allowing muscles to contract naturally and increase in mass, dehydrated muscles will only work to 30 or 35 percent of their capacity. This spells tiredness, aches and pains, headaches, and an inability to build body muscle while losing body fat, which adds more fuel to classic midlife maladies.

Together with proper protein and salt intake, water works to release excess stores of fluid, much like priming a pump. It is *the* natural diuretic. No other beverage works like water to prevent the body from holding excess fluids. Interestingly enough, no other beverage works like water to halt hot flashes; a cool glass of water is often enough to stop a flash in its tracks.

One more thing about the power of water: It is one of the major remedies for vaginal dryness. If you have been looking for a reason to drink more water, here it is, finally: Water is a great lubricant for your *entire* body! Get the eight 8-ounce glasses you need every day—and even more if you are having hot flashes on a regular basis!

Still not convinced? Consider this: Water also works to keep the skin healthy, resilient, and wrinkle-resistant. It could honestly be labeled the first "anti-aging" ingredient!

DRINK YOURSELF WELL

As convinced as we may be about the benefits of drinking water, doing so is a challenge; most Americans have grown up drinking just about anything *but*. We list our favorite beverages as soda, coffee, tea, juice—with water being good only for washing down pills, washing away dirt, and brushing our teeth. Although we often hear that we should drink more water, it's easier to reach for something else. And we pay a price: We miss out on water's benefits.

Even juices and milk contain substances that require the body to process and utilize. With soft drinks, your body has to work especially hard to detoxify and excrete the chemicals and colorings. Although water-based, sodas, teas, and coffees are simply "polluted" water. Many beverages, particularly those that contain caffeine, actually remove more water than is contained in the beverage itself. They act as dehydrators, further increasing rather than fully replacing your fluid needs.

As a matter of fact, each cup of coffee or tea adds an extra cup of water to the eight-to-ten-a-day basic requirement. Who has room—or time—for that many bathroom trips? Coffee, teas, and some sodas contain tannic acid, a product that interferes with iron and calcium absorption and competes for excretion with other bodily waste products such as uric acid. When not properly excreted, this uric acid can build up in the body and crystallize around the joints. This build-up leads to joint pain in elbows, shoulders, knees, and feet, especially former injury spots, and is a type of gouty arthritis. Women in perimenopause are particularly prone to uric acid excesses. This is one reason why a cup of tea or coffee, although fluid based, just doesn't do the job. Water is what those joints are thirsting for; it works to lubricate those midlife achy joints.

HOW MUCH DO I NEED?

Every day you need eight to ten 8-ounce glasses of water—more when you exercise, travel by plane, live at high altitudes, or battle hot flashes. Sound overwhelming? Never thirsty? You're not alone. The water prescription brings out cries of anguish from most everyone who hears it.

Although this water prescription has been recently challenged in the media, you really do need that much because you lose that much every day. Your body continually loses water as it performs necessary functions. Even breathing uses up your fluid stores; every time you exhale, you blow off water—a total of about two cups per day from breathing alone. Water evaporates from your skin to cool your body, even when you aren't aware of sweating. These losses, along with that lost in regular urination and bowel movements, total up to ten cups per day. When perspiring heavily or when experiencing frequent hot flashes, the amount lost can double or triple.

Take heart! As you begin to meet your body's needs by drinking more water, your natural thirst will increase. You may find water drinking habit-forming; the more you drink, the more you want.

Start increasing your intake any way you can: through a straw, in a sports sipper, from a silver pitcher. Add fresh lemon or lime, drink sparkling water, buy bottled water—whatever it takes, just drink it! Try filling a two-quart container with water each morning and then make sure it's all gone before you go to bed. I also encourage a habit of drinking a twelve- to sixteen-ounce glass of water right after each meal and snack throughout the day. If you are eating as often as you should, every three hours or so, this will provide a large proportion of the fluid you need.

TIPS FOR STAYING HYDRATED

Start your day with eight to sixteen ounces of water. While the coffee or tea is brewing, drink a cup or two of water. You wake up with a water deficit, so drinking water soon after arising will gently restore hydration. Many of my clients swear by a cup of warm water with a squeeze of lemon first thing in the morning to jumpstart their digestive system. They declare it the answer to their "regularity" problems.

Get your eight-a-day. Again, this is not a diet principle; it's just how your body is wired. Take water breaks routinely, at least every thirty-five to forty-five minutes, even more frequently when the air is dry or hot or if you are experiencing hot flashes. Drink eight ounces of water before and eight ounces after each meal. Try to drink little or nothing with your meals (sip water if you must), because washing food down with water dilutes the digestive function.

The actual fluid intake formula ideal for you is based on your body weight. An overall guideline is that you should drink a half ounce for every pound you weigh. Thus, for example, a 150-pound person would need 75 ounces (about nine 8-ounce glasses). Although the body attempts to make up any deficit by pulling fluid from the foods you eat, it is preferable to fill the majority of your need with pure, simple water.

Get more when you need it. You may not automatically know when you need more, but look for the subtle signs of dehydration — dry eyes, nose, or mouth, impatience, slight nausea, flushed skin, dizziness, headaches, weakness, and mild fatigue. You may have never related these energy-taxing symptoms to a lack of water. Also, drink more when it's hotter or dryer than normal, if you're more stressed than usual, and when you exercise.

Not to make you obsessive, but it's a good idea to glance at your urine occasionally. Other than first thing in the morning, a dark yellow color is a bad sign, revealing that your kidneys are concentrating their waste in too small a volume of liquid. Pale-colored urine indicates good hydration status.

Don't wait until you're thirsty to drink. It's already too late. Once you feel thirsty, you've already lost a significant amount of fluid. So don't rely on your thirst mechanism. It will prompt you to replace only 35 to 40 percent of your body's hydration needs. And if you don't take in adequate water, your body fluids will be thrown out of balance and you may experience fluid retention, constipation, unexplained weight gain, and a greater malfunction in your natural thirst mechanism.

Keep water where you are. You're more apt to keep up with water needs if you keep drinking water close at hand. Freeze large bottles of water overnight and pull them out in the morning. The water thaws through the day but is still chilled. Keep a glass or a pitcher of water at your desk and refill it often. At home, keep a pitcher or large bottle of water in the refrigerator, with a glass on the counter to serve as a reminder.

Fill up before you work out. Drink sixteen ounces of water fifteen to thirty minutes before your workout. Avoid starting to exercise when you're already thirsty. You're guaranteed a substandard performance if you are low on water before you even begin to move, and you'll have a difficult time recovering.

Continue to fill up while you're working out. Drink six to eight ounces of water every twenty minutes during your workout or training. This may seem like a lot, but even this doesn't begin to keep up with typical sweat losses. When possible, drink cool water—it is absorbed into the system more quickly. No need for a sports drink to replenish electrolytes unless you're exercising longer than ninety minutes.

If you start craving salt, go for water. Once your fluid stores drop below a certain level, your thirst mechanism cuts off altogether (possibly to preserve your sanity if you're lost in the desert?). What turns on is a desire for salt—or for salty foods. It's one of those magnificent things the body was created to do. Because extra sodium holds more fluids in the body, the salt craving is a survival mechanism to slow life-threatening dehydration. Notice a craving for hot dogs and nachos at the beach? Look for a water bottle instead.

IS TAP WATER OKAY?

Be sure not to let the "bottled-versus-tap-versus-treated-water" controversy get in the way of your health. Many people do; they don't trust their tap water, so they drink little of it.

Public water systems today are well monitored for safety, and bottled water companies are now beginning to fall under similar standards. You can assure yourself of the purity and safety of your local drinking water by checking with your local Environmental Protection Agency or health department, or by contacting EPA's Safe Drinking Water Hotline at 1-800-426-4791. If you lack confidence in the answers that you receive, you can also have your water tested privately. The agencies listed above can give you the names of testing laboratories.

If you drink bottled water, choose brands that bottle their water in glass or clear plastic containers and are able and willing to provide an analysis or certification of purity. Buy only spring or purified water; a bottle labeled "drinking water" may just come from your municipal water system. You would do just as well turning on your faucet.

The biggest concern with tap water is that it is treated with chlorine to remove contaminants. As important as chlorine is for purifying our water, I have concerns about it. Thereby, I encourage my clients to attempt to avoid water that has an obvious taste or smell of chlorine.

You may want to get information on a water purifying system for your home if you don't already have one. Steam distillation is the most reliable, and most expensive, form of filtration. The next best is reverse osmosis, which forces the water through a cellophane-like, semi-permeable membrane that acts as a barrier to contaminants like asbestos, copper, lead, mercury, and even some microorganisms. Reverse osmosis systems require a good bit of water pressure to function and are often difficult to access for necessary filter changes. The replacement filters also can be quite expensive.

Activated carbon filters use granules, precoat (a fine powder), or solid block to remove unpleasant odors, colors, and off-tastes from drinking water, and they do a good job in removing chlorine and some contaminants. If all you are after is good taste and less chlorine odor and aren't concerned about microorganisms or other contaminants, a simple tabletop pitcher with a carbon filter (such as Brita) will suffice. If you drink tap water, the taste may improve after refrigerating it for twenty-four hours (some of the chlorine will dissipate). This can be a low-cost way to get the more refreshing taste of bottled water without the cost.

Your choice of which water to drink comes down to taste, cost, and availability. Regardless, the bottom line is this: Don't allow anything to become a substitute for the beverage your body likes best — *water!*

HORMONE BALANCING
ACTION STEPS: WEEK SIX

Drink water—and a lot of it! Ideally, you should drink eight to ten 8-ounce glasses each day.

✔ *Review your diary of last week.* How much water are you drinking on any given day?

✔ *Each day this week, add an extra eight ounces to the water you are already drinking.* Do this until you are up to the amount of water you need, based on the calculation noted above—a half ounce per pound of body weight. Record your water intake in your Food-Feelings-and-Findings Journal. If you drink other beverages that are dehydrating (such as coffee, tea, or soda), add an extra glass of water to make up the healthy difference.

✔ *Continue to choose serotonin-boosting foods for your meals and snacks.* Recall the hormonal balance prescription: Eat early (breakfast within the first half hour of arising), eat often (approximately every 2½ to 3 hours), and eat balanced meals and snacks that contain whole carbohydrates and low-fat proteins.

✔ *Increase walking to thirty minutes, at least five days this week.* If you are doing another form of aerobic exercise, continue to walk on the other days.

✔ *If not every night, choose two nights this week that you will go to bed early enough to get seven to eight hours of sleep.* If you are waking up in the middle of the night, unable to get back to restful sleep, try a bowl of whole-grain cereal and milk as your bedtime snack to stabilize your blood sugars through the night. Also review your day to be sure you are eating evenly.

✔ *Body-spirit balance step.* Choose a special "before bed" relaxer—a warm bath, turning off the electric lights in your bedroom and lighting candles, enjoyable reading, writing down your blessings, a cup of warm decaffeinated tea—for twenty minutes before you say "Good Night." When I end up in bed but am not yet asleep, rather than counting sheep, I recite meaningful Scriptures like this one:

Now may the Lord of peace himself give you peace at all times and in every way.

2 Thessalonians 3:16

Fats:
Friend or Foe?

A re you confused about fat in foods? Do you feel unsure about the good, the bad, and the ugly on this issue? You are not alone; it is likely the most controversial nutrient, with carbohydrates coming in at a close second!

News flash! Not all fat is created equal, nor is all fat bad for you. In fact, fat is an *essential* nutrient, vital for hormone production, vitamin absorption, lubrication, and brain power. Fat should *not* be considered as an "enemy of the state"; it is critical to your health and well-being. But it's important to know which fats are vital to your health and which are not.

For example, essential fatty acids (EFA) are just that—essential for your health. They are the next most important group of foods to be included in the perimenopausal fight, right after phytoestrogens. Essential fats "oil the body" by lubricating the joints, skin, and vagina, as well as serving in many other vital functions, including the production of estrogen.

Without sufficient EFAs, the body will start to send out warnings that there is a deficiency of essential fats. The problem is that these warnings can be subtle at first. Signs include dry skin, lifeless hair, cracked nails, fatigue, dry eyes, lack of motivation, aching joints, difficulty in losing weight, forgetfulness, breast pain—all symptoms that can be confused with perimenopausal ones.

Yet, as healthy as some fats might be, fat also provides the most concentrated source of energy. Even a little can provide a lot of calories. In excess, fat increases the risk of cardiovascular disease, some cancers, and obviously, weight gain. And there are some fats that, in any amount, contribute to body and hormone imbalance.

Generally, we consume five kinds of fat: saturated, hydrogenated (trans-fat), polyunsaturated, monounsaturated, and omega–3 fatty acids. Each contributes the same number of fat grams and calories to the fat budget: five grams of fat and 45 calories per teaspoon. But these fats vary greatly in the effects they have on our bodies—good and bad.

IMBALANCE CAUSES IMBALANCE

The type of fat you consume is equally as important as how much, if not more so. Some fats—namely, saturated and trans-fats—are damaging to the arteries, heart, and brain and appear to increase many perimenopausal symptoms. Other fats, such as the mono-unsaturated and omega–3s, promote wellness. We have to learn to distinguish between the fats we eat rather than choose to cut them out of our diet altogether or to consume fat-laden foods with abandon.

It is the predominance of one type of fat over another in your diet that makes a difference to your health and may explain many of our present-day maladies. This is especially the case when applied to the chemistry of the midlife brain, for fats have a huge impact on its function. Few people realize how critical fatty acids are at the molecular levels of brain cells in fostering clear and rapid message transmission and energy production that keeps the brain function-ing alive and active. It appears that you can take a perfectly good brain and easily confound it by feeding it the wrong type of fat.

A case in point is omega–6 oils. They are the essential oils in nuts and seeds, such as sesame, walnut, sunflower, and soy. They are a source of essential fatty acids and thereby help prevent blood clots and keep the blood thin. They can also reduce inflammation and pain in the joints and are vital in preventing arthritis. All good, right?

Not exactly. The problem with omega–6 oils is their predomi-nance in our twenty-first-century diets. Ample evidence suggests that prior to the Industrial Revolution, we were consuming equal amounts of omega–3 and omega–6 fatty acids, which is perfect for good brain functioning. But today, Americans eat fifteen to twenty times the amount of omega–6 fats as omega–3s, and the result is brain havoc—hormonal and otherwise.

This is because a major issue with hormonal wellness is the body's balance of *prostaglandins*—hormone-like substances that regulate every cell in the body in a multilevel series of complex interactions. When prostaglandins are out of balance, your blood is more likely to clump together, raising your risk of stroke or heart attack. Imbalanced prostaglandins also play a role in cramping, aching joints, and headaches.

One of the easiest ways to get your prostaglandins out of balance and create chronic inflammation is to eat foods that contain hydrogenated oils. Trans-fat is formed through hydrogenation, where vegetable oils are hardened into solids, usually to protect against spoiling and to maintain flavor. Examples include stick margarine and shortening, deep-fried foods such as French fries and fried chicken, pastries, cookies, doughnuts, and crackers. These synthetic oils have the potential to trigger chronic inflammatory responses in

Make a Big Fat Difference!

- Use all fruit jam on toast instead of butter, or use roasted garlic as a spread for hot bread. Warm bread and rolls are always tastier than cold and don't require butter.

- Substitute blended extra-silken tofu or blended-till-smooth, low-fat cottage cheese or ricotta in recipes calling for sour cream or mayonnaise. These products also make a great topping for baked potatoes, especially sprinkled with chives or grated Parmesan, or swirled with salsa.

- Use skim milk, nonfat plain yogurt, part-skim milk cheese, nonfat or low-fat cottage or ricotta cheese and light cream cheese instead of the higher-fat dairy products.

- Eat more fish and white meats and fewer red meats. If you eat red meats, buy lean, trim well (before and after cooking), and cook in a way that diminishes fat, such as grilling or broiling on a rack.

- Use olive oil or cold-pressed canola oil for salads or cooking. You can cut the amount called for in a recipe by two-thirds without sacrificing quality (example: 1 tbs. oil may be cut to 1 tsp. or 3 tbs. down to 1 tbs.); in some recipes, the fat may be cut completely by using nonstick sprays or stock.

- Avoid hydrogenated fat and trans-fats whenever possible; label reading is a must here. Similarly, I vote for reduced-fat or light mayonnaise or dressings — but not fat free, which is often just a chemical brew loaded with sugars.

the brain tissue and muscle because they block the effect of natural oils, which have important and potent regulatory effects on your prostaglandins. Inflammation raises both cortisol and estrogen levels while suppressing progesterone. This, in turn, creates even more stress and more hormone imbalance. Eating trans-fatty acids can also produce a detrimental effect on blood circulation to the brain and its function.

Read the ingredient list of any processed foods you buy. If you see the words "partially hydrogenated," look for a different product—especially if it is one of the first three ingredients.

If I have to make a choice between butter or margarine, I always choose limited amounts of a real food: butter. Buy good quality butter and keep it frozen. If you can't *imagine* bread or potatoes without butter, use just a thin spread and try some of the "fat trimming tips" in the accompanying sidebar.

OMEGA–3 FATTY ACIDS (EPA AND DHA OILS)

The fat your body most needs is omega–3, found in all fish and seafood, particularly cold-water, oily ones such as salmon, albacore tuna, swordfish, sardines, mackerel, and shellfish.

Omega–3s are also present to some extent in pumpkin seeds, walnuts, dark green vegetables—with flaxseed being the only significant plant source. They serve to directly fight the maladies of menopause, combating depression, increasing lubrication, boosting brain power, softening the skin, and improving energy levels. These special fats also reduce the risk of heart disease and decrease triglycerides and LDL cholesterol while increasing HDL cholesterol. In addition, they reduce the tendency of the blood to form clots, stabilize blood sugars and blood pressure, and reduce inflammation.

Without omega–3s, brain cells do not function at optimal levels. This oil tells your brain to feel good. It serves as

High Omega-3 Recipes	
Terrific Tuna Grill	300
Chicken of the Sea Sandwich	305
Seared Shrimp with Edamame, Corn, and Tomato Saute	310
Poached Salmon over Black Bean, Corn, and Edamame Salsa	319
Snapper with Tomato and Feta Cheese	320

a mood elevator, even in the midst of depression. Moreover, these oils can increase your metabolic rate and serve as a natural diuretic through increasing production of prostaglandins that enable your kidneys to eliminate excess fluids.

FINDING FISH

I strongly recommend fish and seafood as a source of protein and for the healthy type of fat it provides. Virtually all fish contains some heart-protective, health-enhancing omega–3 fatty acids, and population studies around the world show health benefits from eating fish of all kinds. I plan my weekly meals to include three to four servings—enough to keep the body healthy and the brain happy, working toward hormone balance.

The fish with the most omega–3 fatty acids, however, are oily, cold-water varieties like salmon, trout, tuna, kippers, mackerel, and sardines (see the High Omega-3 Recipes). When possible, go for wild salmon, which has a significantly higher omega–3 content than farm-raised salmon.

About fish safety: There is no other type of food in which freshness and purity is so critical. Know your "fishmonger"; find out when the fish comes in and buy on those days. Really fresh seafood should smell faintly of the sea but sweet. It should not be offensively rank or have a "fishy," ammonia-like smell.

Because almost all shrimp is frozen immediately after being caught, I ask for two- or five-pound bags, still frozen, and defrost only what I need, when I need it.

If you do not want to eat fish, there are some vegetarian sources of omega–3 fatty acids, notably flaxseed.

OIL WITH A DIFFERENCE: FLAXSEED

Flaxseed has taken center stage in health these days—with good reason, specifically related to its impact on menopausal symptoms. Flaxseed is similar to soy with its range of benefits. Flaxseeds are unusual in that they contain not only the omega–6 oils that other seeds contain, but they also contain good quantities of omega–3 oils that typically only come from fish and seafood. As a matter of fact, flaxseed is the only significant plant source of omega–3—a definite plus for the woman who *doesn't* love fish!

Flaxseed also contains the same "good" prostaglandins found in fish oils, so it may be helpful in regulating other perimenopausal symptoms, such as excessive menstrual bleeding.

As you read in chapter 21, flaxseeds are also rich in phytoestrogens but of a different type than soy—lignans as compared to isoflavones. Flaxseed is packed with these lignans, and when we eat them, they are converted in the intestines to an estrogenic compound. Lignans may also share estrogen receptor sites, regulating the effects of this estrogen dominance. In addition, a high lignan intake has been associated with lower incidence of cancer, along with significant brain-boosting power.

Two tablespoons of flaxseed is estimated to be the equivalent of one portion of soy in terms of phytoestrogens. I suggest using both soy and flaxseed—if not together, interchangeably. It will expose you to a variety of phytoestrogens to obtain the best results.

Flaxseeds are small—about the size of sesame seeds—so they are very easy to mix with other foods. Buy them whole at a natural-food store and keep in the refrigerator. You may want to "grind to order" in a pepper mill or grind a half cup or so at a time in a blender or coffee grinder. Ground flax has a nutty taste that is delicious mixed into yogurt or into power shakes, and they are great sprinkled on breads, rice, cereals, or salads.

In addition to the flaxseeds themselves, you will see dark plastic bottles of flaxseed oil in the refrigerated case of the natural foods store. I don't advise using it over flaxseed—the oil oxidizes readily and easily develops an unpleasant taste. Furthermore, although flaxseed oil contains the omega–3s, it does *not* contain phytoestrogens, so it is ineffective for hormonal impact. Opt for the ground flaxseed instead.

Seed Mix

Making and using a "seed mix" is a delicious and effective way to receive the beneficial qualities of essential fatty acids as well as phytoestrogens. I make a blend of one part each sesame, sunflower, and pumpkin seeds, mixed with two parts flaxseed. Store the mix in a sealed container in the fridge and, as with flaxseed alone, lightly grind the quantity you need for a week, using a coffee grinder apparatus, and store the rest in the fridge.

There is some research indicating that taking supplements containing large amounts of the so-called good oils, such as those found in borage oil, evening primrose oil, and flaxseed oil, can relieve the inflammation and discomfort that comes with a headache or PMS, much as taking an aspirin will relieve pain. I do recommend these to many of my clients. However, because we only need EFAs in the very tiny amounts found in fish, nuts and seeds, whole grains, and fruits and vegetables, using the relatively huge amounts of the EFAs found in the supplements may not be warranted as a first step, and are certainly not my first line of treatment.

Recipes with Flaxseed	
Breakfast Shake	296
Hot Apple-Cinnamon Oatmeal	298
Seeded Tortilla Triangles	308

KNOWING NUTS

Nuts and seeds, although a source of fat, are wonderfully nutritious additions to your pantry. Use sparingly (because of their calories) and take care with buying and storing them (because of their fragile nature). As with most healthy ingredients, fresh is king—the naturally occurring oils in nuts and seeds can quickly go rancid.

Buy only fresh nuts and seeds, stored air-tight, well within the "use by" date. Store them in the refrigerator or freezer and check them regularly for freshness. Rancidity is usually detectable by your nose or taste buds. Sniff first and throw out any products that develop an off smell.

MONOUNSATURATED FATS

Monounsaturated fats, such as olive, canola, and peanut oil, are considered heart healthy, working to increase good HDL cholesterol and decrease bad LDL cholesterol. But these valuable oils actually do much more for the body than protect the heart.

Olive oil is the star monounsaturated fat. It works to protect the brain and prevent memory loss and decline in cognitive function. Researchers suggest that similar to fish oil, olive oil helps to maintain the structural integrity of the brain. In addition, olive oil is power-packed with phytochemicals that work as antioxidants in the body, combating aging and brain-cell damage. It's the oil of choice for cooking because there is less chance of creating aging free radicals.

When it comes to getting the most benefit from olive oils, quality counts. Look for cold-pressed extra-virgin olive oil, which is made traditionally from whole, ripe, undamaged olives. This type of oil has not lost any significant phytochemical activity through processing.

I use small amounts of healthy and flavorful monounsaturated extra virgin olive oil for most all of my cooking. Some chefs prefer to use a lower quality olive oil for certain cooking techniques—such as frying—but since I do no frying and use only a small amount of oil in any dish, the extra virgin variety is always my choice. I do use a less expensive one for cooking and a more exquisite one for finishing dishes, especially for salads.

For the few recipes that don't take well to the flavor of olive oil, such as banana bread or muffins, I used cold-pressed canola oil, another monounsaturated fat. It's not as highly refined as the classic canola oil but typically requires a trip to the natural foods store to find it. I also use a drizzle of flavorful sesame oil and walnut oil for certain special recipes, though never for cooking; they do not stand up well to heat.

Oils should be purchased in small bottles and kept tightly closed in a cool, dimly lit spot in your kitchen or pantry. Exposure to light and air can oxidize the oil, which makes it susceptible to attack by free radicals (linked to premature aging and cancer). I store good oils in the refrigerator, warming the bottle in running hot water before using.

Is your head spinning from all these facts on fat? Let me boil it down to a simple bottom line. Try to get most of your fat from monounsaturated olive and cold-pressed canola oil (or salad dressings made from them), nuts, and the omega-3s found in fish and flaxseed. And spread your fat throughout the day—a little fat helps you absorb fat-soluble nutrients from vegetables and fruit.

Recipes with Monounsaturated Fats	
Trail Mix	165
Nut Butter Danish	299

Focus on smart fats. Use moderate amounts of extra-virgin olive oil, canola oil, and nuts as your main added fat and increase your intake of omega–3 fatty acids through fish and flaxseed. Avoid hydrogenated and trans-fats.

✔ *Review your diary of last week.* Circle the foods that you suspect may contain hydrogenated and trans-fats, and red-star those that contain smart fats — the omega–3s (such as fish, seafood, and flaxseed) and monounsaturated fats (such as olive oil).

✔ *Plan your meals for this week to up the ante on smart fats.* Begin eating some fish if you do not already do so. Salmon is easily available fresh, so it may be your best place to start. If you are not a fish eater, look at the ways you might add flaxseed into your daily diet. If you have not used extra virgin olive oil before, now is the week to begin.

✔ *Go through your pantry and refrigerator and aggressively evaluate the foods within them for their type of fat.* Box up and donate unopened packages of foods that are heavy on hydrogenated and trans-fats; make a grocery list for picking up smart fats, such as olive oil and flaxseed. You may need to make a trip to the natural foods store to find flaxseed. (While you are there, pick up a bottle of cold-pressed canola oil and store it in the refrigerator.)

✔ *Check the mileage you are walking in your thirty minutes.* If you are walking less than two miles, pick up your pace a bit. Continue walking at least five days a week.

✔ *Body-spirit balance step.* Do a fun activity outdoors, weather permitting. Even if it's a cloudy day, you'll receive the benefit of sunlight and a boost by having a good time! It may be biking, a trip to the beach, volleyball, canoeing, gardening, or walking down to buy flowers. You'll soon learn about why this is such a power move for your hormonal balance. As you do, be on the lookout for examples of how God's creation is intricately designed to nourish every living thing. The sunlight nourishes plants, which in turn nourish us.

Walk while you have the light.
John 12:35

THE
CALCIUM CURE

With all the buzz about our increasing risk of osteoporosis, you may be wondering if you are getting enough calcium to stay strong in midlife. But just how much *is* enough? It's an important question, because reduced estrogen levels *can* lead to significant bone loss.

As we've already identified, the decision to take estrogen is a thorny one, but those who do opt for Hormone Replacement Therapy are often encouraged to begin as soon as possible in order to minimize bone loss in the interim. However, on the osteoporosis front, there are a number of alternatives to HRT. This chapter will help you to personally evaluate them and identify your first and healthiest choice.

Getting proper levels of calcium is certainly number one. Recent research suggests that this bone-building mineral provides many health benefits beyond simply strengthening bones. Among perimenopausal women, these include fewer bothersome symptoms as well as reduced blood pressure, lowered colon cancer risk, and better weight management. In a recent study, menstruating women who received 1,200 mg of calcium per day had significantly less intense symptoms of PMS, and some had no symptoms at all.

In another small study conducted at the University of Tennessee, researchers found that the more dietary calcium the study group consumed, the less body fat they produced. The theory is that when short on calcium, the body produces a hormone called *calcitrol*, which encourages the body to store fat and fat cells to become bigger and better. When adequate calcium is received, the body sends a message to the fat cell to burn fat for energy—excellent news for people in midlife!

Before age thirty-five, women should consume at least 1,000 mg of calcium a day. That's roughly equivalent to the amount of calcium in three eight-ounce glasses of skim milk. Women over thirty-five should get 1,200 mg a day, and menopausal women should get upwards of 1500 mg. Unfortunately, few women in any category get enough. The more at risk you are for osteoporosis, the more calcium you need.

A recent U.S. study of more than 200,000 postmenopausal women ages fifty and older, published in the December 2001 issue of the *Journal of the American Medical Association*, found that nearly half had thinning bones and did not know it.

As we all know, milk and other dairy products are excellent sources of calcium. But this building mineral is found in many foods, and these days food producers are adding it to everything from orange juice to breakfast cereal. There are many calcium-rich foods, and a varied diet of these will make a wonderful difference. Your best bet is to get calcium from several sources. Here are some choices and what they can provide for you:

> 1 c. milk = 300 mg
> 1 c. of low-fat, plain yogurt = 447 mg
> ½ c. skimmed milk ricotta = 335 mg
> 1 c. of tofu (with calcium sulfate) = 408 mg
> 1 c. calcium-enriched orange juice = 300 mg
> 1 c. of cooked collard greens = 355 mg
> ½ c. of canned salmon = 284 mg
> 1 oz. low-fat cheese = 200–270 mg
> ½ c. whole almonds = 156 mg
> 1 c. cooked or 2 cups raw broccoli = 200 mg
> 1 c. cooked beans = 95–130 mg
> 1 oz. fortified breakfast cereal = 250 mg per serving

LACTOSE INTOLERANT?

It's estimated that nearly fifty million Americans are lactose intolerant—meaning that they produce too little lactase (the enzyme that digests lactose, the naturally occurring sugar in milk products). The symptoms are bloating, gas, cramping, and diarrhea. Some women are genetically inclined to be lactose intolerant, others increasingly become so as they proceed through midlife and perhaps experience some intestinal changes. This leads many women to skip dairy products altogether. However, because these products are great sources of calcium, learning how to skip the bloat but not the calcium is in order.

Some dairy products such as yogurt (with live cultures), buttermilk, and cheeses contain less lactose, so will be better tolerated. You can also buy lactase in a pill form (such as lactaid) and can use lactose-reduced milk. In addition, you can use calcium-fortified soy products, such as soy milk, soy cheese, soy yogurt, or tofu; they are all lactose free.

CALCIUM SUPPLEMENTS?

If you suspect that your calcium intake is lacking, you may want to consider taking a calcium supplement. I recommend brands that contain synthetic calcium. Calcium derived from bone meal, oyster shells, or another natural source is sometimes contaminated with lead.

The least costly calcium supplements are those containing calcium carbonate. These products, including Tums and Caltrate, are not well absorbed, so they are best taken with meals. If it's more convenient for you to take calcium between meals, consider paying a bit more for Citracal or another supplement that contains calcium citrate, by far the most absorbable form of calcium.

Whatever the source of calcium (food or supplement),

High Calcium Recipes	
Baked Breakfast Apple	295
Breakfast Shake	296
Ricotta Breakfast Sundae	296
Toasted Cheese and Pears	297
Hot Oatcakes	297
Hot Apple-Cinnamon Oatmeal	298
Terrific Tuna Grill	300
Hot Carrot-Cheese Melt	301
Swiss Stuffed Potatoes	301
Grilled Turkey and Cheese Sandwich	304
Tuscan Broccoli	314
Snapper with Tomato and Feta Cheese	320
Spaghetti Pie	321

the body is able to absorb only about 500 mg at a time. Given this constraint, it's smart to spread your calcium intake out over the day. Do not exceed 2,500 mg of calcium daily, as an overdose can cause fatigue and metabolic disturbances. Having a glass of calcium-fortified orange juice with breakfast is fine, but a half carton after a workout is probably too much!

ABOUT VITAMIN D

To make sure that the calcium you do consume is properly absorbed, keep careful watch over your intake of vitamin D. You can get all the vitamin D you need by going outdoors in sunlight without sunscreen for fifteen minutes a day; unprotected skin makes its own vitamin D when exposed to sunlight. If you're prone to skin damage from the sun's ultraviolet rays, you can take a vitamin D supplement. (Milk also is fortified with vitamin D.) I recommend 400 international units (IU) of vitamin D a day for sun-deprived women over thirty-five.

Don't forget about the rest of your diet when it comes to getting the most use from your calcium intake. Too much caffeine, sodium, or phosphates (found in soft drinks) can leach calcium from the body. Too much protein *blocks* calcium absorption—a serious concern given America's ongoing fascination with trendy high-protein diets.

If avoiding osteoporosis is your primary goal, remember that bones are affected by more than just how much calcium you get.

> **Did You Know?**
>
> If you've seen the headlines that "sunshine may prevent cancer," you probably wonder if the world isn't going crazy. Sun exposure causes skin cancer, so how can this be? There is indeed some research showing that a small amount of sun exposure may reduce the risk of certain cancers, as well as help keep bones strong. Scientists have found that mortality rates for some cancers — notably breast, colon, ovarian, and prostate — tend to be lower in sunnier regions. And some studies have found that people who get little or no sun exposure tend to have higher rates of breast and colon cancer. Why? Since sunlight's ultraviolet-B radiation is responsible for producing vitamin D in the body, researchers have wondered if this could be the connection.

Regular exercise—especially walking, jogging, dancing, and other weight-bearing activities—builds bone. Good eating and good exercise always pop up as the dynamic duo for wellness!

HORMONE BALANCING
ACTION STEPS: WEEK EIGHT

Get plenty of calcium-rich food!

- ✔ *Review your diary of last week.* Count the number of calcium-rich foods you consumed each day, consulting page 216 for help. Red-star the days that you consumed at least four servings from food. If you consumed less, go to the next step.

- ✔ *Look for high calcium alternatives to your food choices that could help make up the healthy difference.* Or, alternatively, decide to supplement with calcium citrate at bedtime, and begin to do so this week. Keep your calcium supplement by your toothbrush, where you'll be reminded to take it. At the end of each day, review the calcium-rich sources you did eat and supplement with 500 mg if you took in less than three servings and 1,000 mg if you took in one or less. Resolve to go for more tomorrow.

- ✔ *Evaluate your diary for calcium robbers, such as soda, coffee, and tea.* Think through alternatives to those beverages. Revisit your water intake and be sure you are consuming at least eight to ten 8-ounce glasses each day.

- ✔ *Try for variety in your power snacks and breakfasts.* Refer to the recipes index in this chapter for some fresh ideas, particularly noting those high in calcium.

- ✔ *Body-spirit balance step.* Pepper your days this week with small pleasures. Every little thing you do gives you an immediate mood boost. Take a walk in the park, spend time in the garden, concentrate on a hobby, or take time off to spend an afternoon with someone special. Whatever you do, try to get outdoors for at least twenty minutes each day. The vitamin D production that comes through the sunlight exposure is invaluable. Lift up your eyes and know that the sun is shining on you!

You created my inmost being;
you knit me together in my mother's womb.
I praise you because I am fearfully and wonderfully made;
your works are wonderful,
I know that full well . . . .
All the days ordained for me
were written in your book
before one of them came to be.

Psalm 139:13–16

TAME THE TANTRUM WITH WHOLE GRAINS AND FIBER

As you have read, carbohydrates are the premium fuel choice for the brain. Eating whole carbohydrates throughout your day ensures your body the energy it can use. And this is where whole grains come in; they are a foundational component of the Hormone Balancing Plan, working to help keep your blood sugar and serotonin levels up and even.

Foods made with refined grains, such as white bread, white pasta, and white rice, are digested quickly and are speeded into the bloodstream as sugar. As positive of a boost as this may seem to be for a moment, the rapid breakdown triggers a flood of insulin, the hormone that ferries the sugar into the cells. Shortly thereafter, blood sugar levels drop precipitously, which signals a release of other chemicals bent on raising blood sugars, among them adrenaline, one of the stress hormones that produces the fight-or-flight response in a panic situation. With it, the adrenal glands release cortisol, bringing with it a flood of distress—and often a hot flash as well.

I know it's unfair. After all, the only thing you ate was a bowl of frozen yogurt a couple of hours ago, and here you are with sirens blaring, red lights flashing, the jitters, racing heartbeat, cold sweats, and anxiety.

By contrast, brown rice, oats, and whole grain cereals take much longer to digest. So insulin levels rise gradually, blood sugar levels remain steady, and cortisol levels don't skyrocket. The brain is fueled, not dive-bombed. You've prevented a sugar crash in the first place, which is a much saner approach—and a critical one for hormone balance.

As you read in chapter 19, our blood sugar level is one of the more powerful influences on our well-being, our ability to lose weight, and our appetite. From a chemical perspective, regulating our blood sugar level is our most effective move for stabilizing serotonin production. It's not hard to even out the blood sugar seesaw when eating early, often, and balanced. Taking care with the type of carbohydrates you eat will take you further still to fine-tuning your body for an even flow of feel-good chemicals.

THE ENERGY RELEASE RATE OF FOODS

Everyone responds poorly to a high glucose load, but some respond worse than others, based on their sugar sensitivity. Moreover, some foods trigger a faster blood sugar rise than others, based on how quickly the food's energy is released into your system. Some foods will raise blood sugar levels dramatically and quickly (fast release), others more moderately (quick release), and some just a little (slow release). The rate of this release is called *glycemic response.*

When the glycemic response is high and the resulting blood sugar rise is fast, the insulin released into the bloodstream is abundant. The high insulin level will outlast the sugar burst, taking more and more sugar into the cells and dramatically dropping the blood sugar levels to a less than desirable level. The result is you may soon feel spacey, unable to concentrate, weak, sleepy, anxious, or dizzy. The quick drop in blood sugar can also trigger cravings for more carbohydrates. In addition, the higher levels of circulating insulin stimulate the storage of fat in the cells and inhibit the burning of fat as energy. This is why eating evenly and wisely will keep blood sugars and insulin levels in check and enable your body to burn fat and release optimal energy.

Most of the popular diet plans and books written in the past decade have addressed this issue of the hormonal and blood sugar response to food and attempted to solve it in different ways. Sadly, the attempts are most always knee-jerk reactions causing pendulum swings. Many diets prescribe cutting out *all* carbohydrates, but this is not the answer, because all carbohydrates are not the problem. It's our typically unbalanced diets that are wreaking havoc: refined carbohydrates eaten to excess. The key to long-term wellness and hormone balance is to get plenty of carbohydrates, but to make them "whole" and not to overload.

SLOW RELEASE "FRIENDLY" CARBOHYDRATES

Some foods result in a lower insulin surge than others and are considered smart choices for day-by-day eating, especially for those seeking stable blood sugars and lower insulin levels.

Beyond their provision of energy and stabilizing impact on blood sugars, whole grain carbohydrates are particularly valuable because they have not had the outer layers of grain removed; they contain many more vitamins, minerals, and fiber than the refined, white products. When you eat whole grains, you receive the blessing of vitamin B6, selenium, magnesium, and folic acid. As you've read, these nutrients are particularly helpful in stabilizing and soothing brain chemical and hormone production. White, refined grains

Better Choice Grains	Better Choice Legumes	Better Choice Vegetables	Better Choice Fruits
oats	chick peas	carrots	apples
barley	kidney beans	corn	apricots, dried
buckwheat	lentils	green peas	small bananas
bulgar or cracked wheat	navy beans	lima beans	cherries
Uncle Sam's Cereal	soybeans	sweet potatoes	grapefruit
Kellogg's BranBuds with psyllium	soy foods	yams	grapes
long grain brown or basmati rice	peanuts		kiwis
quinoa			mangos
spelt			oranges
whole wheat couscous			peaches
whole wheat tortillas			pears
whole wheat or artichoke pasta			plums
100% stoneground whole wheat bread			tomatoes
whole grain pumpernickel bread			
whole wheat sourdough bread			

have been stripped of these nutrients in the manufacturing process (forty-one nutrients are forever lost through refinement).

Don't be fooled by manufacturers and advertisements. White, refined carbohydrates, even when enriched, are never as good nutritionally as whole grains. In fact, to your body, refined white flour is the same as sugar, making a diet high in white flour foods the same as a high-sugar diet. Start reading the ingredients lists of all your grain products and remember to choose the ones made with 100 percent whole grain (with the word "whole" listed first). Many manufacturers call products whole grain even if they contain only minimal amounts of bran. Brown dye does wonders in making food look healthy!

BUYING THE BASICS

Stock up on whole wheat or artichoke pastas and brown rice; they are chewier and more filling than their white flour counterparts and are a nice alternative. The same goes for other grains, such as amaranth, barley, cracked wheat, whole wheat couscous, quinoa, and spelt.

High Fiber Recipes

Baked Breakfast Apple	295
Hot Oatcakes	297
Hot Apple-Cinnamon Oatmeal	298
Nut Butter Danish	299
Seeded Tortilla Triangles	308
Marinated Tempeh with Broccoli and Red Peppers	311
Chili Con Tofu	312
Brown Rice Pilaf	314
Stir-Fried Tofu with Asparagus and Shitakes	315
Chicken Pad Thai	316
BBQ Grilled Tempeh Sandwiches with Chopped Tomato Salad	317 – 18
Spaghetti Pie	321

BULK UP WITH FIBER

Whole grains satisfy and keep you full. One of the reasons for their satiety value is the fiber they contain. There are two types of fiber: the water-soluble fibers found in oats, barley, apples, dried beans, and nuts, which have been found to lower serum cholesterol and triglyceride levels and to help control blood sugar levels; and the water-insoluble fibers found in wheat bran, whole grains, and fresh vegetables, which are an excellent means of controlling chronic gastrointestinal problems.

Think of fiber as a sponge that absorbs excess water in the GI tract to curtail diarrhea but provides a bulky mass that will pass more quickly and easily to relieve constipation and diverticulosis, as well as possibly prevent hemorrhoids. Fiber needs water to make it work the way it should—the eight to ten 8-ounce glasses a day you are working toward!

When choosing carbohydrates, go for the most whole form possible and thus benefit from all the fiber, nutrients, and natural chemicals they were created with. This means eating fruits and vegetables with well-washed skins on, and choosing fruit more often than fruit juice. Choose whole grains when you can, such as brown rice and stoneground, 100 percent whole grain breads, crackers, pastas, and cereals (again, the word "whole" should be the first ingredient). Look for a variety of whole-grain English muffins, small-sized bagels, tortillas, pitas, and crackers. Your natural foods store is most apt to have 100 percent whole grain choices. Cereals should have less than five grams of added sugar, excluding that from any dried fruit it may contain.

Foods High in Fiber

- peanuts and peanut butter
- cooked dried beans
- sunflower and sesame seeds
- apples, apricots, peaches, pears, bananas, pineapple, plums, prunes
- broccoli, carrots, corn, lettuce, peas, potatoes (including skins), spinach
- bran (unprocessed wheat and oat)
- bread (whole wheat)
- brown rice
- cereals: whole grain, bran type, oatmeal, wheatena
- whole wheat pasta

HORMONE BALANCING
ACTION STEPS: WEEK NINE

Use whole grains for their phytochemical, vitamin, and mineral protectors and wealth of blood sugar stabilizing fiber.

✔ *Continue to choose foods for your power meals and snacks that provide for stable blood chemistries.* Review your diary for food choices that may contribute to better stabilization. For example, you may need to choose more of the best-choice whole grains and legumes on page 223, balancing them with low-fat proteins. Also, evaluate the timing of your power snacks and meals. Are you eating infrequently or often?

✔ *Look for ways to increase your fiber intake.* You may want to add ground flaxseed, unprocessed oat, and/or wheat bran to your cereal, salads, or power shakes. Be sure to get plenty of water as well in order to activate that good fiber for your body.

✔ *Experiment with the meal ideas and recipes I have provided.* Break out of your rut! Add pizzazz by selecting at least three new recipes you intend to try this week.

✔ *Go through your pantry once again.* As you do so, make a shopping list for the whole grain varieties of carbohydrates to replace those that are refined. Box up unopened packages and donate to your food pantry.

✔ *Check the mileage you are walking in your thirty minutes.* If you are walking less than two miles, pick up your pace a bit. Continue walking at least five days a week.

✔ *Body-spirit balance step.* Shake things up! You probably have a suitcase full of habits and ruts that you aren't even aware of. Becoming conscious of these routines (your journal will help!) and then breaking and altering them will give you a different point of view, reminding you that you are in control of your choices and can change things. It can do a world of good for your well-being because it breaks you out of the slump of entrapment.

Consider moving the furniture. Mix up your schedule of doing things in the morning. Do your work in a different location. Eat a different breakfast. Listen to some new music. Take a different route today. You may want to reflect on this declaration and receive strength for change:

> *Forget the former things;*
> *do not dwell on the past.*
> *See, I am doing a new thing!*
> *Now it springs up; do you not perceive it?*
> *I am making a way in the desert*
> *and streams in the wasteland.*
>
> Isaiah 43:18–19

Kick the Habit: The Sugar and Caffeine Blues

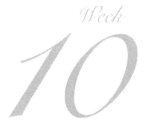

So now you know what to eat in order to dramatically improve your quality of life through perimenopause and beyond. But what are the foods *not* to eat, that is, those that will dramatically worsen bothersome symptoms? Truly, there are foods that can add to the misery factor—generally those that serve as inflammatory agents or central nervous system stimulants.

If you asked me to give you a prescription guaranteed to bring on hormonal imbalance, it would be to eat erratically and eat plenty of high-calorie, high-sugar foods made with refined carbohydrates and hydrogenated or unsaturated vegetable oils. As you've read in chapter 23, trans-fatty acids (partially hydrogenated oils) block the good anti-inflammatory prostaglandins, and refined sugar and caffeine stimulate adrenaline, cortisol, and insulin production, all of which contribute to blocking progesterone effectiveness and raising cortisol levels.

If you want to achieve hormonal balance, avoid these foods. Let me remind you once again: The mainstay of this meal plan is plenty of fresh vegetables and whole fresh fruits, whole grains, lean meats, fish, and lots of water.

REFINED FOODS AND SUGARS

Compare labels of fat-free treats with their full-fat versions, and you are likely to find that, in many cases, the calories of fat-free foods are as high or actually higher. That's because sugar and other quickly digested simple carbohydrates are used to make up for the fat-based ingredients. Getting your blood sugar off track can boomerang by making you hungrier in a little while.

When blood glucose levels fall, your body releases adrenaline from the adrenal glands. Constantly signaling the adrenals into action can lead to adrenal exhaustion—bad news for perimenopause, since the adrenal glands serve to produce a form of estrogen when your ovaries start producing less.

Although most often the object of cravings, these substances trigger a response like throwing gas on the fire of hormone-charged symptoms. Refined sugars have been shown to aggravate just about every symptom of PMS and to have a dramatic effect on one specific menopausal complaint: postmenopausal vaginitis. You read about the potential for dry and thinning vaginal tissue in chapter 12. Eating too much sugar or allowing blood sugars to stay high (as in the case of poorly controlled diabetes) can create an alkaline environment in the vagina, which may leave the vagina more susceptible to the bacteria that contribute to vaginitis.

So what's the bottom line on refined sugar in perimenopause and beyond? Avoid it as much as possible. It does your body little good and can do it considerable harm, particularly in large doses. The good news is that sugar is an acquired taste—the more you eat, the more you will want, and the less you eat, the less you will want. You will experience fewer energy drops and mood swings as well.

One of the biggest blunders we make in eating isn't about eating at all. It's not just the taste of sweets that tickles our fancy and flames the fire of desire; it's about depending on food for a chemical brain boost to get us through the rough times when energy is low and we're being dealt some tough blows. The two prime examples of substances to which we give too much power are sugar and caffeine. Let's take a look at breaking the grip of them both.

JUST A SPOON FULL OF SUGAR . . .

As we have noted, a heavy sugar intake brings a pleasurable rise in feel-good brain chemicals, which will be followed by a quick fall a few hours later. That dip often triggers "eating for a lift" to relieve the resulting fatigue, brain fog, and mood drop. Usually the chosen food is again high in sugar, and the seesaw effect continues. Then the guilt tapes begin to play: *You've already blown it, so go ahead and finish the cookies before you get "back" to healthy eating.* And the more you eat, the more you crave, trying to get that same boost.

Equalizing your brain chemistries is a key to balancing hormones because too-low levels of serotonin and endorphin trigger the craving for a drug that will provide fuel for these neurotransmitters. Of course, not everyone is as sugar sensitive as some; not everyone turns a bite of chocolate into an addictive drug. But there is ample evidence that some folks can use sweet foods and refined carbohydrates as powerful mood-altering drugs — and experience the similar roller coaster of behavior and thoughts of an addict.

People without such an inflammatory chemical response will experience a pleasurable feeling from the rise in brain chemicals that follows the eating of refined carbohydrates and sweets. But people with a heightened sensitivity will experience a powerful euphoria — not just feeling good, but *great!* These folks can be trapped in a vicious cycle of highs and lows controlled by soaring and plummeting body chemistries. Even those who violently oppose drinking or the use of street drugs can get on a different path of addiction; alcohol may not hook them, but sugar, ice cream, chocolate, and soda do.

And the dependency on such substances can be just as strong. In fact, if you have used alcohol or drugs in an addictive way at some time in your life, it's likely that you have a body chemistry that responds more intensely to these chemicals than other people. This body chemistry doesn't change in sobriety; it often just finds another "drug of choice," and that can be sweets.

How much sugar do Americans consume? We now eat the equivalent of about 31 teaspoons of added sugars per day, on average. That's 500 calories' worth or about 20 percent of our total calorie intake. That includes sugars added by manufacturers to foods like soda, flavored yogurts, and cookies as well as those added directly by the consumer, such as what we add to iced tea or spoon on cereals. How much weight will you lose in one year if you just cut that added sugar in half, with no other changes? Twenty six pounds for an average adult.

If sugar is affecting your well-being, make it your goal to cut back on your daily use of sweets and other refined carbs and eat whole carbohydrates and fruits to stabilize your body chemistries and satisfy your natural craving for sugar. I would certainly question whether sweets are worth robbing yourself of your precious energy and stamina!

With that said, let me also warn you against setting up sweets as a "forbidden fruit." Iron-fisted discipline and will power can crumble when faced with a simple piece of chocolate. It didn't work for Eve and the apple, and it won't work for you. What *does* work is accepting the realities and consequences of our choices—and choosing instead to "feast" on the fruit that brings life!

For help in kicking the sugar habit, use the following tips.

Know your enemy. Sugar is called by many names: honey, brown sugar, corn syrup, fructose, and so on. But it's all sugar! Much of our problem with sugar lies in the fact that it is hidden in nearly every packaged product on the grocer's shelf.

Be very careful if sugar (or any other name for sugar, such as any word ending in–ose) is in the top three ingredients in a packaged product. If it is, you're getting more than you are bargaining for! And, as you've read, sugar resides in refined carbohydrates that have been stripped of their fibers and nutrients, allowing a quick "rush" into your bloodstream.

Know yourself. How much is enough for you, and how much triggers the desire for more? Does nibbling a little bit of sweets lead to a lot? It does for many women who find that even occasionally eating high-sugar foods is difficult, for the seesaw effect results in a "the more you have, the more you want" syndrome.

If this sounds familiar, it may be necessary for you to "just say no" to sugar-laden foods for long enough (twelve to fourteen days) to allow your blood sugar and brain chemical levels to stabilize and to allow your energy and appetite for healthy foods to return. Only then can you assess the impact sweets have on your body—and your resolve.

Know that withdrawal is real. If you are sugar sensitive, you are apt to experience physical symptoms of drug deprivation. You may feel shaky, nauseous, or edgy, or you may experience headaches or diarrhea.

As you embark on any healthy lifestyle change—especially as chemically impacting as pulling back from a high intake of sugar—your body needs time to adjust physiologically and emotionally. It will take at least five to six days before the change begins to feel comfortable physically. You can expect the following:

- Days 1 and 2: You may feel slightly sluggish, irritable, and dissatisfied with your eating.
- Day 3: This will be one of your most difficult days as your body begins to feel the chemical change. It may seem that every cell in your body is crying out for food, particularly something sweet. Expect this day to be a struggle, but not one impossible to overcome.
- Day 4: If you make it through the third day without overeating or killing someone, this one won't be so difficult!
- Day 5: This may be a day of a ravenous appetite; you can expect to be hungry for food—not sweets necessarily, just food. You can eat a meal and still think: *That was a good appetizer—what else is there to eat?*
- Days 6 and 7: By now it should be getting easier and easier; you have more energy, and you have more control over your appetite. You are now on the road to a lifetime of good eating! The surprise of feeling good makes it all worth the effort.

I know these symptoms may sound more like withdrawal from hard drugs than simply allowing your body to adjust to a wonderfully healthy way of eating. But let's face reality: Putting in healthy foods means leaving out the unhealthy, and that means a chemical change—a withdrawal of sorts. You need to know what to expect. If you recognize that the chemical changes are a temporary but necessary part of establishing new eating patterns, it will be easier for you to break through to a lifetime of good eating. You will have the strength to speak back to cravings and appetite and choose instead to eat nourishing, healthy foods.

Know when you're vulnerable. Identify and avoid resolve-breakers like fatigue, hunger, anger, or loneliness. They are often the music playing in the background of temptation! If your life response has been to eat when you're tired, to "get through," it is more difficult to choose to break for a nap than to reach for cookies. If you have spent a lifetime pushing down anger with food, it is more difficult to choose to journal your anger or discuss its cause when you are furious. Frenzied eating feels more natural, and food is always oh-so-accessible!

Know the drill. Resist the "I've already blown it" syndrome! Even when you succumb to temptation and consume foods you know interfere with your health, be assured that a lapse in healthy eating doesn't ruin all the health you have attained over weeks of wellness. A lapse in your healthy lifestyle is just that—a lapse. Don't let it become a relapse, another relapse, and finally a collapse. Look at each meal and snack as an event; don't wrap it all into one bad day or one unhealthy weekend. Instead, get right back on track with the next meal or snack. Your body will stabilize quickly, you'll feel great, and you'll be thanking yourself the next day!

Know that it will get easier. A baby is born with a natural preference toward foods with a slightly sweet taste in order to draw him or her to breast milk. But these taste bud preferences become overdeveloped and fueled by a lifetime of high sugar intake and erratic eating patterns, now drawing us to highly sweetened foods. As you cut back, over time, your cravings will diminish and your taste buds regain their ability to pick up the sweetness in a carrot or piece of fruit.

Power snack throughout the day. Just in case it hasn't sunk in yet, eating every two to three hours throughout the day keeps your energy okay and a ravenous appetite away! Go for energy-boosting combos like fresh fruit or a box of raisins with low-fat cheese or yogurt, a half sandwich, or a trail mix of dry roasted peanuts and sunflower seeds mixed with dried fruit. Keep power snacks available wherever you are; they will serve as a lift to your body and prevent the drowsiness and sweet cravings that often follow meals.

Rely on the natural sweet treat. Fruit is the natural fulfillment of our sweet desires. And remember to go for the fruit, not the fruit juice; the fiber slows the release of the fruit's simple carbohydrate, which prevents blood sugar spikes and insulin surges.

Consume enough fiber. Remember that the water-soluble fibers found in oats, barley, brown rice, apples, dried beans, and nuts serve as a "time-release capsule," releasing sugars from these digested carbohydrates slowly and evenly into the bloodstream. This helps keep your energy levels up and even and your cravings down.

Save sugars for last. If you do have sweets, add a dessert onto the end of a meal rather than having the treat *as* your meal or snack. This allows the balanced meal to temper the insulin surge, keeping blood sugars more stable.

WHAT ABOUT ALCOHOL?

You may have watched it on *60 Minutes*, or you may have read about it in the newspaper. It's called "the French paradox," and it's all about wine, particularly red wine, being good for you. You read that a moderate amount of alcohol, in any form, actually extends life and may help to offset the negative health effects of a high fat diet. Your friend's cardiologist recommended that she drink a glass of Merlot every night to raise her HDL cholesterol; it would be good for her.

But is it true? And, if so, how does that advice fit into the Hormone Balancing Plan?

It is true that a moderate intake of alcohol has been found to have positive health benefits, and the research is strong and promising enough to result in many physicians recommending a daily glass of wine to their patients.

But it is also true that, over time, excessive alcohol can result in a chronic energy drain. Its impact on your blood sugars increases your appetite, interferes with your sleep, and robs you of the absorption and function of many of the energy nutrients. The extra calories it adds to your intake can contribute to weight gain or prevent weight loss. And more than moderate intakes can damage your internal organs (such as your liver, intestines, and heart) and increase risk of cancer, particularly that of the liver and breast.

The medical benefits of wine or other spirits are just not compelling enough to encourage people who don't drink to begin just to get those benefits. The U.S. Dietary Guidelines say this: "If you drink, do so in moderation—and don't drink and drive." What is moderation? For women, it's considered to be a four- to six-ounce glass of wine, a light beer, or one and a half ounces of liquor a day. Because of the impact on your blood sugars, it's best to fit this into your meal plan as a simple carbohydrate, substituting it for one of your pieces of fruit at a meal.

How about a refreshing mineral water and lime instead?

WHAT ABOUT ARTIFICIAL SWEETENERS?

As you become aware (and possibly alarmed!) about your intake of sugar, you may be tempted to make the switch to sugar substitutes. *Don't!* There are no absolutes in the safety of chemicals — saccharin (Sweet n' Low), aspartame (Nutrasweet or Equal), sucrolose (Splenda), or any new one to come along. The long-term effects of their use will not be known for years.

For example, in the years since Nutrasweet has appeared on the market, cautions concerning its use have accelerated. Questions have been posed about its allergic reaction in some, its impact on brain chemistry because of its crossing the blood barrier of the brain, its danger with possible breakdown in hot foods, its effect on children and the unborn, and its connection to the rise in brain tumor incidence. The verdict is not in.

That battle will continue, for although aspartame and other sweeteners are made from "natural" sources, they are still chemically produced in a laboratory and are not found in nature. The possibility for future problems to result from frequent use is real. Concerns have been raised about the potential of Nutrasweet to hinder the brain's formation of serotonin, causing the let-down that follows aspartame intake to bring anxiety and depression along with an increased appetite. That may be why a recent Tufts University study showed that drinks containing aspartame, saccharin, or Acesulfame K increased the desire to eat and reduced feelings of fullness.

Also consider that aspartame is made from phenylalanine, which is an amino acid. High doses of a single amino acid can throw off the balance of amino acids in your brain and body. Because phenylalanine is a precursor to dopamine and norepinephrine, which are stimulating neurotransmitters, high usage of aspartame can create a "speed-like" effect.

There is also concern about aspartame's potential to keep insulin levels elevated, thereby heightening disease risk and adding to the obesity problem. Remember, foods alone don't make insulin rise; just the sight, smell, and taste of food can do so. But in the case of artificially sweetened beverages, there are no calories for the insulin to work with, so the blood sugar level drops, stimulating hunger.

Finally, understand that as long as you continue to use sugar-laden foods or sugar substitutes, you will keep your taste buds trained for sugar. The goal is to cut back on its use so you no longer need everything to taste overly sweet. Allow your taste buds to change so that the desire for sweetness can be met in a safe way—from fruits and other naturally sweet foods that are healthy outlets for our inborn sweet preference.

How about you? Do you have a sweet that seems to call your name? If chocolate is your sugar seductress, you may be hooked on more than the sugar alone. In addition to the chemical impact of chocolate on the brain's neurotransmitters (research shows it to release similar substances as those released in romantic love), chocolate packs a one-two punch with a double hit of sugar *and* caffeine. Not so different from that double mocha-cappucino that may woo you in mid-afternoon! Or maybe it's that caffeine/aspartame-pumped diet soda—the equivalent of rocket fuel to many.

> ### Additives, Preservatives, and Other Chemicals
>
> Try to buy your food in the most natural state possible. Even though additives, preservatives, and flavorings are used in small quantities in manufactured foods, if a large percentage of your diet is based on processed foods, you will amass all the small amounts in all the different products you eat and drink every day. Over a period of time, these small amounts add up, and a chemical cocktail is created within each of us. Nobody knows exactly how these chemicals will react together. Your body has to deal with them somehow, resulting in energy and vital nutrients being spent when they could be used for more profitable ends, such as disease prevention and hormonal balance.

TEA, COFFEE, AND SODAS

So, what's wrong with tea, coffee, and soda? For starters, tannic acid, which interferes with the absorption of minerals and the excretion of other waste products, like uric acid. Then there's the caffeine issue, which serves as yet another central nervous system stimulant to spark hot flashes and place a strain on the adrenal glands as well as further disrupting sleep.

In small doses, caffeine can be an effective pick-me-up, producing clearer thinking, sharper sensory awareness, and a quicker reaction time. Like other drugs, however, there is a downside to caffeine: Too much causes a surge of adrenaline. But when the spurt is over, power levels plummet and stress hormones are produced. Studies have shown that the stress hormones are still circulating—and elevating blood pressure—up to eight hours after the last caffeine hit. And those stress hormones play a key role in disrupting hormone production and function. Combine this impact with the blocking action these hormones play on serotonin production, and it's not surprising that caffeine can also aggravate PMS and mood swings in women.

If you are experiencing hot flashes, any amount of caffeine can be too much by causing constriction or tightening of the blood vessels in the skin. Caffeine can elevate body temperature, cause high blood pressure, and possibly trigger the flash itself. Even small amounts of caffeine may cause side effects, including restlessness and disturbed sleep, heart palpitations, stomach irritation, and diarrhea. It can promote irritability, anxiety, and depression. Furthermore, caffeine is a diuretic and can flush out and deplete the body of many vital nutrients and trace elements such as vitamin C, several B vitamins, calcium, potassium, and zinc—all needed in perimenopause and beyond. All the while it adds to the dehydration plaguing most midlifers.

There are also substances in caffeinated drinks and foods (such as chocolate) called methylxanthines, which have been linked to a benign breast disease called fibrocystic disease. This condition makes the breasts feel more

Teas That Please

These simple, aromatic, and delicious teas are immediately invigorating.

Lemon-Rose Tea

½ tsp. dried rosemary

½ tsp. dried lemon balm

Boiling water

Steep for 10 minutes in a cup of boiling water, covered. Strain, and sweeten with 1 tsp. honey, if desired.

Ginger Tea

½ tsp. grated fresh ginger root
   (peeled and grated lengthwise
   on the large holes of a grater)

Boiling water

½ tsp. honey, or to taste

Put the ginger into a cup of boiling water, cover, and let it steep for 10 – 15 minutes. Strain, add honey to taste, and drink hot or iced.

uncomfortable, tender, and lumpy in the few weeks before your period begins; this phenomenon worsens as you approach menopause when estrogen is fluctuating wildly.

Swollen and tender breasts can add to already difficult sleep and, quite clearly, can impact intimacy. Interestingly, the problem can often be eliminated simply by cutting out coffee, chocolate, cola drinks, cocoa, and tea. Just switching to the decaffeinated versions doesn't necessarily help because methylxanthines are found in the decaf versions as well.

Good warm beverage alternatives for coffee and teas are readily available. You might try herbal teas, fruit teas, and decaffeinated green tea. If you switch, be sure that you drink any beverage in moderation. They still don't give the benefits of water.

Green tea is a particularly interesting drink. Both green and "ordinary" black tea come from the same plant, but in green tea the leaves are not fermented, thereby retaining more of its polyphenols, a particularly potent antioxidant. I usually suggest that my clients who are big coffee drinkers try to switch to caffeinated green tea as a first step in their coffee withdrawal; it reduces the caffeine concentration and gives some healthy benefits to boot.

Of course, the best alternative of all is pure wonderful water—the more, the better!

ARE YOU A JAVA JUNKIE?

Do you need to cut out caffeine altogether? Not necessarily. Despite its drawbacks, it's definitely an energy booster. My concern is when caffeine becomes your best friend. I do encourage you to cut back slowly to a ceiling of 250 mg, which is the amount at which the stimulant effect—and most of the negatives—of caffeine kicks in. This is the amount in one mug of brewed coffee or three glasses of iced tea. If, after cutting back to this amount, you still experience any of the above-mentioned effects of caffeine, particularly hot flashes and fibrocystic issues, I would suggest withdrawing altogether. You'll also get more of an energy boost from the caffeine you do consume if you have cut back on your intake.

Because caffeine is also found in soda (regular and diet), chocolate, and even decongestant cold pills, it adds up quickly. And the levels soar when you get java from a gourmet coffee shop. Analysis shows that these specialty brews can contain two to three times the caffeine found in a cup made from your typical supermarket brands. These specialty coffees are stronger because more grounds are used to give the brew its rich flavor, making the coffee even more potent. In fact, one large cup of specialty coffee packs a walloping 280 mg of caffeine, and some have been reported at 550 mg. At these higher levels of intake, about 600 mg, you can get *too* energized and start to feel the java jitters: frazzled nerves, the shakes, insomnia, and ultimately, fatigue.

REAL WITHDRAWAL

Pain is the word that best characterizes cutting back on caffeine consumption, and that is why you must do so gradually. Again, caffeine is a powerfully addictive drug, which will bring withdrawal symptoms as you give it up. Many people experience zombie-like fatigue, irritability, lethargy, and headaches from going "cold turkey." These symptoms may last for up to five days. People expect to feel better from doing such a noble thing as giving up espresso but end up feeling horrible instead. Then they drag back to caffeine, positive they can't live without it.

If you determine it is wise to cut back on your caffeine intake, do so *slowly* over the course of a week to ten days. Start the withdrawal process by cutting back to a safer level of two cups of coffee or three glasses of tea. Gradually cut back, a quarter of a cup at a time, until you are down to none. Or substitute a decaffeinated product for the real thing in the same reducing amounts.

Withdrawal will be less painful if you follow the Hormone Balancing Meal Plan. Eating small, balanced meals throughout the day will stabilize your body chemistries and reduce your reliance on caffeine for energy. Note that if you focus on drinking more water than you have in the past, you won't have room for the other beverages! In addition, try to get outdoor exercise every day to get a boost of feel-good endorphins. You'll read more about that in chapter 27.

Finally, whether it's a mindset you want to break or the grip of sugar or caffeine, don't set up any food as a forbidden fruit. There are no good or bad foods; there is no such thing as a legal or a cheat food. Food is simply food. The power it lords over us is the problem. While it's important to assess the physiological power that eating may have over our body chemistries and develop a better plan, setting our focus on what we shouldn't do and what we shouldn't eat only sets us up for failure. Our eyes become so fixed on the negative behavior or food that it becomes an obsession. Then it's only a matter of time before we fall headfirst right into it.

Instead, set your eyes on what *to* do — choosing foods that nourish and energize you, bringing a sense of peace and calm to your body.

HORMONE BALANCING
ACTION STEPS: WEEK TEN

Reduce your intake of stimulants, such as refined sugars and caffeine.

✔ *Review your food journal to assess how many sweet-laden or refined carbohydrate foods you consumed on any given day.* Note any correlation between your food choices and your feelings, emotionally and physically. Were you more apt to have a sweet when you were down or fatigued, or up and celebrating? Did eating the sweet result in any increase in bothersome symptoms later? What were those?

✔ *For each sweet-laden food event, look at the other options that may have been available.* Determine other choices you can make in the future.

✔ *Look at your beverage choices and do the math.* If one cup of coffee or three glasses of iced tea or soda will each give approximately 250 mg of caffeine, how much caffeine are you consuming on average in a given day? How much water do you drink? Do you see an increase in bothersome symptoms with a higher intake of caffeinated beverages? Are there substitutes that would work for you?

✔ *Go through your pantry once again, this time looking for foods containing high amounts of sugar (-ose in the first three ingredients).* Add a variety of fresh or frozen fruits to this week's grocery list, as well as a few different Japanese or Chinese green teas to try. If you drink coffee or black tea, try to substitute green tea for some or all of your usual beverages—or try the lemon-rose or ginger tea on page 238.

✔ *Increase your walking to forty minutes, five days a week.*

✔ *Body-spirit balance step.* Give yourself permission this week not to be perfect. Inside all of us is the kid we used to be—the kid who didn't have to be perfect and worry about everything (or shouldn't have had to!). Give yourself a break. Place a photo of yourself as a child in your bedroom or at your desk at work so you can see it each day, and remember to nurture yourself and laugh. Thank God for all he has done to nurture you from that young child into who you are today. Spend time with children as well; they are wonderful reminders of how playful and fun life is meant to be.

Therefore we do not lose heart . . . inwardly we are being renewed day by day. . . . So we fix our eyes not on what is seen, but on what is unseen. For what is seen is temporary, but what is unseen is eternal.

2 Corinthians 4:16, 18

EXERCISE
YOUR OPTIONS

Okay, it's clear—perimenopause may be natural, but it's surely a shock to the system. And it's made more difficult still by our unnatural, sedentary lifestyles.

Whatever the effects of your shifting hormones—the fat gravitating toward your abdomen, hot flashes, anxiety, depression, declining energy, poor sleep, declining self-esteem, problems with memory and concentration—there is one thing that can boost your mood, melt away fat, and improve almost every aspect of your health picture. No, it's not a $49.95 infomercial special; it's exercise! Consistent, moderate, balanced exercise, combined with strategic eating, is the second part of the dynamic duo for hormone wellness. A little bit of walking, toning, and stretching goes a long way toward improving the overall quality of your life—now through menopause.

As an example, let's look at some research on exercise and hot flashes. One study of more than 1,600 women found that sedentary women were twice as likely to report hot flashes as physically active women. Another study reported a drop in the incidence of hot flashes immediately following a forty-five-minute aerobic workout.

VALUES OF EXERCISE

Exercise has the amazing ability to restore your energy level, regardless of whether you are suffering from fatigue, anxiety, or depression. It will calm and soothe you. And the good news is that you feel energy and mood-altering benefits the instant you start to exercise.

That's not all. Lacing up your sneakers is virtually a call to action for the hormones that reverse fat storage and process out stress. Other studies have proven the effectiveness of exercise for stabilizing mood disturbances and insomnia as well as reducing the physical stress response.

Because of the interconnected nature of the muscular system, brain, and other processes of the body, being sedentary depresses your mood, your thinking, and your ability to work productively. But moderate regular exercise can create a change in that biochemistry, launching you into a state of confidence and exhilaration and boosting your energy, moods, and alertness. There's strong evidence that moderate exercise—a brisk walk, a forty-five-minute strength workout—also triggers the release of the "pleasure chemicals" known as endorphins. In addition, working up a good sweat activates the "feel good" neurotransmitters dopamine and serotonin, which, as you've learned, reduce the intensity of just about every perimenopausal symptom. It can tame even the worst case of PMS!

Regular aerobic exercise such as walking also increases your circulation, which helps to minimize bloating and fluid retention. It definitely impacts hot flashes, possibly because of its impact on circulation and cooling or because of the accompanying endorphin release. Exercise also decreases your appetite and gives you a healthy outlet for stress—it douses the emotional fires behind overeating.

Finally, your muscles are loaded with insulin receptors. The more muscle mass you have and the more heat you generate from your muscles on a regular basis, the more efficiently you'll use insulin and burn body fat, overriding the midlife message to "store, store, store"! We know that what most influences weight gain in midlife is not hormonal status alone but the loss of muscle mass and the accompanying decrease in metabolism. Exercise—specifically strength training—reverses the reduction in metabolic rate while simultaneously increasing muscle mass. Furthermore, research shows that you can accomplish this goal at any age.

The overall effect of consistent exercise is to provide you better fuel to work with and a better engine to put it in.

I've been exercising, in one form or another, for a long, long time, although I didn't always know it. I didn't call it exercise in my teens; I called it *dancing!* I was on my high school's Rockette-like dance team, which required two to three hours of practice a day. And I danced every weekend night for hours at a time (or until my curfew came!).

It never occurred to me that my love of dancing was providing me with something my adolescent, hormonally shifting body desperately needed: exercise, movement, stress release, serotonin boosting. I now know that with my roller coaster emotions, poor teenage eating habits, and yo-yo dieting, exercise may have been the stabilizing force that kept me relatively balanced and my parents somewhat sane!

When I entered into the study of nutrition, all of my focus went to my eating patterns, optimizing them and nourishing my body with the best of food at the best of times. I was freed from a ten-year captivity of yo-yo dieting and lost weight naturally. I also started consistently walking or running.

And I have been doing so—every day—for about twenty-five years now. I've used it as my reflective time and prayer time when I'm alone and as valuable communication time when I walked with my husband. Always for more than just burning a few calories, my daily exercise worked to boost my metabolism and emotions out of a lifetime dieting trap and genetic proclivity to being overweight. It has been a hormone stabilizer and bone strengthener—and a powerful stress release.

But then I turned forty-five, and sadly, it became apparent that walking alone, although a great exercise, was no longer enough for this overstressed, over-forty body. I had to face that it wasn't giving me the overall bodybuilding and toning I needed to face midlife changes with strength and resolve.

MY AHA MOMENT

You see, I really didn't want to take supplemental hormones if I could do without them. A couple summers ago, as I was in the very throes of hormonal change, I came to the awesome realization that as important a role as eating well was to stabilizing my hormones, I was going to be chopped liver if I didn't significantly step up my whole exercise experience.

If you are just starting out with exercise, simply walking can work wonders for your body and your hormonal state; hopefully, you have already begun to realize its benefits these past few weeks. But I had been well conditioned aerobically through my years of dancing, running, and walking—so much so that my daily walks were barely raising my heart rate, my metabolism, or my fat-burning capacity. Although I did a bit of conditioning, my free-weight routine frequently lost out to time pressures. It was erratic and non-specific, so I was slowly losing lean body muscle. At the same time, my hormone levels were swinging wide and low, and the necessary transition of estrogen production moving to my fat cells was occurring seemingly at warp speed.

Even though my eating was, obviously, excellent in the nutritional arena, I was laying down bigger and better fat cells right through my abdominal area, hence the change in body shape. And because I had been thin for many years, my midsection fat cells were very, very hungry!

What did I need to do? Embrace exercise with a renewed passion and vigor. I knew exactly what to do in the nutritional arena to stabilize my brain chemistries and to provide hormonal balance—the very Hormone Balancing Meal Plan you've been reading about. It was now time to apply my knowledge to the area of exercise, specifically strength training. More than just needing to "take it up a notch," a well-rounded workout needed to become as strong a focus as eating well. That choice has helped to make my past year—and my body response to hormonal change—much different from the preceding ones in my own perimenopausal crossing.

This is primarily because of the impact that focused exercise has on muscle mass. When you start *using* muscle during exercise rather than *losing* it to midlife, you release your fat-burning potential. Strong muscles are a lot like the Energizer Bunny: They just keep going and going, activating your metabolism and revving up the body's calorie burning ability, even while you sleep.

This is why exercise, particularly strength training, together with positive nutrition, is the anti-aging solution. Lifting weights curbs muscle loss, along with shaping a sleeker, firmer body. Weight-bearing exercise such as walking or weight lifting also promotes bone growth—a big plus in the battle against osteoporosis. And if you build up to walking at a brisk clip (4 mph), you may encourage your body to secrete more growth hormone, which both strengthens bones and increases lean body mass.

MY PERSONAL EXERCISE PRESCRIPTION?

I joined the local Y. I bought a heart rate monitor. I began to run-walk for forty-five to sixty minutes, six days a week on the treadmill or through the neighborhood, varying my speed (and when on the treadmill, the incline) based on keeping my heart rate in my target zone of 130 to 150.

I do a twenty- to thirty-minute strength-training workout on Mondays, Wednesdays, and Fridays, and I do a stretching routine on Tuesdays and Thursdays. On Sundays, I take a long, relaxing walk or bike ride—just because.

Sure, it takes a lot more time than it used to. Because of that, I don't get to follow through perfectly with my plan every single day, every single week. And that's okay; yet when I do get to do so, I feel the difference, and I like it.

I believe that exercise is a vital part of my anti-aging and menopause-without-HRT solution, and I would encourage it to be yours as well. My personal revelation has been confirmed again and again in research. Miriam Nelson's landmark Tufts research (which you can find in her book *Strong Women, Stay Young*, Bantam, 1997) scientifically proved that by incorporating just two strength-training sessions per week into their lives, women could actually reverse the effects of aging and hormone decline. After one year of strength training in the Tufts program, women's bodies were fifteen to twenty years more youthful. Without drugs or hormones, they regained bone, helping to prevent osteoporosis. They became stronger—in most cases, stronger than when they were younger. They lost fat and built muscle, becoming leaner and trimmer without dieting. What's more, the women were so energized that they became 27 percent more active.

"JUST DO IT!"

Why *don't* people exercise? I believe the answer is simple: Too many of us are stuck in a vicious cycle of exhaustion. We know we need to exercise, but we are simply too done in to get it done. That's why I usually develop a phased exercise plan for my clients, first getting them eating well and encouraging easy walking. You see this reflected in this Hormone Balancing Plan. After a few weeks, a more focused exercise strategy emerges as a result of the overflow of new energy. With this dynamic duo, the exercise adds significantly to their level of well-being, and a positive cycle replaces the negative, downward energy cycle.

When you feel too tired to "just do it," keep reminding yourself of this: *The fastest way to feel energized is to exercise.* That "I'm too tired to work out" feeling will get out of your head once you start moving. You just have to override the message of your stressed-out brain and do something—anything—physical when you're in an energy slump. When you get home feeling totally beat, push yourself a bit. Change into sneakers and go out for a brisk walk. You'll feel a burst of energy afterward. Then the next time you're feeling too pooped to exercise, you'll remember that "buzz" and be quicker to get off the couch. You may even be inclined to expand your workout into a more ambitious run or bike ride or even a visit to the gym. Soon you'll be healthfully hooked on the buzz of working out and won't even hear those "I'm just too tired" messages from your brain.

The best motivation for exercise in midlife is embracing the knowledge that exercise will *neutralize* perimenopausal symptoms, including hot flashes—pure and simple. But here is a review of top ten reasons to exercise, motivators to get you on a path for focused exercise and strength training.

1. *You'll improve your overall well-being—period.* The boost of serotonin that results from an exercise session is just the boost your hormone-strapped body needs, enhancing mood, outlook, energy, and sleep.
2. *You'll turn back the clock.* Women who complete even one year of strength training have been found to appear to be fifteen or twenty years younger than when they began.

3. *You'll build bone mass.* Weight-bearing exercise such as walking or weight lifting promotes bone growth—a big plus in the battle against osteoporosis.

4. *You'll slim your middle.* Those who exercise regularly have been found to not experience the age-related decline in their resting metabolic rate as do their sedentary counterparts, so they stay thinner and healthier, longer.

5. *You'll get a good night's sleep.* A Stanford University study of forty-three men and women with mild insomnia revealed that those who walked briskly for thirty to forty minutes four times a week for four months slept almost an hour longer per night and fell asleep faster.

6. *You'll look better.* Regular exercise gets your blood moving as well as your body. This increased circulation transports nutrients to your skin and quickly flushes out waste products. This leaves your skin glowing with enhanced health.

7. *You'll substantially reduce your risk of breast cancer, diabetes, heart disease, and osteoporosis.* A Harvard University study found that women runners have half the risk of developing breast cancer that sedentary women do. Regular physical activity is associated with reduced blood pressure, an increase in good cholesterol and reduction in bad cholesterol, reduced total body fat, weight loss or maintenance of ideal body weight, and improved handling of sugars in the blood. In more global terms, a number of studies have shown that higher activity and/or fitness levels are associated with dramatically lower rates of cardiovascular disease, diabetes, and certain cancers.

8. *You'll take stress in stride.* When you're confronted with a stressful situation, your body prepares to fight or take flight, in part by secreting catecholamines, chemicals that raise your heart rate and blood pressure and pump blood to large muscles in your legs and arms. Your fight-or-flight response then "burns off" those calories. The problem is this: You most often don't have the option to fight or flee, yet your body is still releasing catecholamines that it doesn't use up. Moreover, your heart rate and blood pressure, as well as your stress level, remain elevated. The best way to get rid of those chemicals? Simulate the fight or flight: walk, run, or hit tennis balls.

9. *You'll be a more creative thinker.* According to many recent studies, regular aerobic exercise can improve your memory, enhance your imagination, and make you more creative. The right side of your brain — that area specializing in creative thought and problem solving — becomes more active when you exercise. It ignites your ability to solve problems, thrive under pressure, and perform at peak levels of effectiveness. As you dramatically increase your oxygen uptake as well as the production of the red corpuscles that carry oxygen to your brain, the influx of blood oxygen enhances the functioning of every organ in your body. Your thinking power receives a forceful boost because 25 percent of your blood is in your brain at any one time during exercise.

10. *You'll protect yourself against diseases of aging.* Researchers at the Harvard School of Public Health found that a thirty-minute brisk walk or jog cut the risk of colon cancer in half. Physicians at Case Western Reserve University and University Hospital of Cleveland report that a history of regular exercise seems to reduce the risk of developing Alzheimer's. Exercise enhances your immune system and generally improves the functioning of almost every organ and system in your body. One study found that those who walked briskly for forty-five minutes a day, five times a week, had half as many colds and bouts with the flu as nonexercisers.

If you continue to struggle with the motivation to get up and get moving, consider joining a fitness center. The pluses are many; I attribute my consistency and diligence with exercise this past year to joining my local Y. Here are some of the reasons.

- *You are not alone.* Other people provide companionship, advice, and encouragement.
- *You can strength-train on machines along with free weights.* Machines are designed to get you into the right position for a move. This means you can isolate the muscle you're working without having to pay quite as much attention to the rest of your body.
- *Other equipment or classes are available.* You might enjoy using treadmills, stair climbers, or elliptical trainers — or try Pilates

or step aerobics. Anything that encourages you to become more active is the goal.

- *Instruction is usually available.* A certified fitness trainer can fine-tune your workouts and get you past any rough spots.

NO PAIN, NO GAIN?

The notion of "no pain, no gain" is an exercise lie. If you hurt, you'll stop exercising or get hurt, and the benefits of activity will come screeching to a halt. The key with exercise is to not let it become a stress. Too much, too hard—two to three hours of hammering the body—zaps energy. Moderation in all things, even exercise, is the age-old word of wisdom.

Before beginning or increasing physical activity, you should take some precautions to ensure a healthy start. To avoid soreness and injury, start out slowly and gradually build up to the desired amount to give your body time to adjust. Most healthy individuals can safely start a light to moderate exercise program without much concern.

However, if you have chronic health problems or symptoms that suggest them, such as heart or lung disease, diabetes, asthma, or obesity, you should first consult your doctor before increasing your level of physical activity.

At the very least, you may want to begin your exercise program with a fitness physical, which can be performed by your doctor or wellness professional. An ideal fitness physical is an "all points check" testing the following: cholesterol, EKG stress test, VO2 max, fat/lean body composition, blood pressure, and resting heart rate. This battery of tests helps you to evaluate if there are any potential risk factors in your

Lose Twice as Many Pounds

Researchers at the University of Pittsburgh School of Medicine found that women who exercised for at least 150 minutes a week (that's 30 minutes five times a week) lost nearly twice as many pounds — 25 versus 14 — as women who exercised less. Losing weight and keeping it off may require more exercise than previously thought — maybe as much as an hour each day, according to this new research.

In another study from Brown University, researchers found that 2,500 people who lost an average of 60 pounds and kept it off for a year exercised about an hour a day. Most of the people in this study walked about ten miles a week, then did aerobics, weight lifting, or other activities.

planned exercise program as well as to set realistic goals. It's a terrific benchmark for beginning and can be very motivating.

Fitness is most easily understood by examining its components, so let's design a well-rounded workout for you. Basically, four types of exercise are needed to provide the best workout and to work all the muscles of your body: warm-up and cool down, aerobic exercise, conditioning and strength exercise, and stretching for flexibility.

WARM UP AND COOL DOWN

Use warm-up exercises, such as light side-to-side movements, to limber up your muscles and prevent injuries from the other types of exercise. Never skip the warm-up; it prepares your muscles for the workout (muscles work best when they're warmer than normal body temperature). A warm-up also allows your oxygen supply to ready itself for what is to come, alerting your body to oncoming shock or stress.

You can warm up with stretching, jumping jacks, skipping rope, or jogging in place. You can also warm up with stretching and then begin a less intense version of your exercise activity—for example, walking before jogging. An adequate warm-up time is three to five minutes.

At the end of your exercise time, also spend three to five minutes cooling down. This allows your body's cardiovascular system to return to normal gradually, preferably over a ten- to fifteen-minute period. This can be considered a "warm-up-in-reverse" because it consists of the same types of exercises as your warm-up.

Warm-up and cool-down are just as important as the main event. Both can prevent many of the common injuries that take you out of the race.

AEROBIC EXERCISE

I recommend thirty minutes of moderate activity, such as brisk walking or bicycling, at least five times a week for fitness and hormone balance. Or, forty-five to sixty minutes of moderate activity at least five times a week for weight loss and increased muscle mass.

When doing aerobic exercise, it's a good idea to keep track of your heart rate. This is especially important when you are building up to a pace and distance that's ideal for you.

How high should your heart rate climb? Assuming you are a healthy individual, an ideal aerobic exercise session should include a warm-up period for five to ten minutes, an endurance phase for thirty-five to forty-five minutes, and a cool-down phase for five to ten minutes. During the endurance phase, the target heart rate should be 70 to 85 percent of your maximal heart rate.

Your maximal heart rate can be estimated by subtracting your age from 220. If you are fifty years of age, your maximal heart rate is 170 and your target heart rate is 119 to 146 beats per minute. In this zone, your muscles are moving, you're breathing deeply, your blood is delivering ample amounts of oxygen to your body systems, and you're burning fat as your major fuel source. At this level, you should be breathing deeply but comfortably enough that you could hold a conversation or sing to yourself.

When you begin your exercise program, aim for the lower part of your heart rate target zone (60 percent) during the first few months. As you get into better shape, gradually build up to the higher part of your target zone (75 percent).

To see if you are within your exercise heart rate zone, take your pulse periodically throughout your exercise time. Place the first two fingers of your hand at either side of your neck just under your jaw. You should feel your pulse easily at your carotid artery. Using your watch or the clock, count for six seconds, then multiply by ten. This is your heart rate per minute.

A fun way to determine whether you are exercising within your ideal zone is to buy a pulse meter, a gadget worn on the wrist or chest that monitors heart rate. It works great for those who have a difficult time mastering the art of checking their heart rate while continuing to exercise. My heart rate monitor has absolutely been the best investment I've made in exercise this year, for it has enabled me to take charge of my exercise time. I can stay so focused on keeping my heart rate in the right zone that the time passes quickly.

If you don't exercise hard enough to get your heart rate up into your target zone, you won't produce the body and brain changes that fully boost your metabolism, energy level, and mood. However, exercising harder than your target heart rate is self-defeating; it can diminish the effectiveness of your workout. Working to such elevated levels causes you to burn more glucose as an energy source, detracting from fat loss and the conditioning of your body. It can also leave you feeling exhausted rather than exhilarated.

No time? Break up your workouts into shorter bouts throughout the day. Reports show that squeezing in even ten-minute spurts of activity throughout the day yields results. Take advantage of the humdrum tasks that have to be done anyway. Haul the garbage cans to the curb yourself; rejoice when you carry that laundry basket up and down the stairs and vacuum with vigor! Even though regularly scheduled aerobic exercise is best for losing fat, any extra movement boosts the metabolism to better burn calories. Start parking at the far end of the lot or make several trips up and down stairs instead of using the elevator.

CONDITIONING AND STRENGTH: LIFT WEIGHTS

Muscles are your calorie-burning furnace, so the better you maintain them, the higher you keep your metabolic rate. Weight training is essential for women over forty to compensate for the decreased muscle mass from falling hormones.

Conditioning or strength exercises are those that tone, shape, and define the muscles through repetitive movement against resistance. Conditioning increases muscle strength and mass by putting more than the usual amount of strain on a muscle, which stimulates the growth of small force-generating proteins inside each muscle cell. These proteins feed the "fibers" that grow during exercise. When you make muscles work harder, you actually tear these fibers. As they rebuild, they get stronger and bigger, resulting in harder, tighter, and more defined muscles.

Strong *and* Happy!

To maximize exercise's mood-boosting power, combine aerobic activity and strength training. After reviewing thirty-two studies on activity and mood, researchers found that a combination of low-intensity aerobic exercise (such as walking or cycling) plus strength training just two to three days a week left people feeling much happier.

Conditioning exercises activate the metabolism by making demands on the muscles that change their chemistry, making them more energy efficient.

Not only does exercise help you to better burn the calories you take in; it also serves to build muscle mass. One more time—that's the midlife weight management secret: In order to rev up your metabolism and burn fat, use—don't lose—your muscle. Building new muscle through strength training is one of the best ways to reverse the metabolic slowdown of midlife and stressful living. And since calories are burned primarily in your muscle, maintaining muscle mass is a key factor in helping maintain a healthful weight. The more lean muscle mass you can preserve, the bigger "engine" you'll have in which to burn calories.

Resistance training has a beneficial effect on your body composition. From about age twenty on, sedentary women lose 1 percent of their muscle mass each year. By age forty, it's 20 percent. Between the ages of twenty and sixty, inactive people can lose up to 40 percent of their muscle mass. And the flabbier muscles are, the less muscle fuel (energy) they can store. That means less strength and stamina for you. By the age of forty, up to a half pound of muscle—and the energy stocked inside—is generally replaced with a half pound of fat.

By reversing this process, weight training can see you through midlife with the energy, strength, and metabolism you had at twenty. As your muscles grow and become more active, the level of energy within the muscles increases, making you more vital. In addition, stronger muscles offer more support to your joints, pump up your sports performance, improve your balance, and help prevent injuries. And regular weight training exercises can boost your cardiovascular health by improving your levels of good cholesterol (HDL). Resistance training also strengthens your bones and helps increase bone mineral mass to help prevent osteoporosis.

Here's a note from Beverly, a new believer in the power of exercise:

> I have been working out two years with a trainer. When we switched to doing a total body conditioning and strength workout twice a week (with two classes of yoga ball, for a total of four mornings a week), my cholesterol dropped to 175-from 239-with an increase in my HDLs from 60 to 74.This is a miracle!!! I have

been in the 239 range for at least 15 years and never dreamed that focused exercise could make such a difference—especially in a mature woman of 65!

A conditioning or resistance workout usually involves various exercises that focus on different muscle groups. This is the essence of circuit training on machines like Nautilus, which were built for this purpose. Normally the exerciser does one to two "sets" of each exercise (a set can be anywhere from eight to fifteen repetitions and takes about one minute to complete). A typical session lasts about thirty minutes. But any kind of repetitive resistance training is effective, whether it's circuit training on weight machines, an arm workout with three- to five-pound free weights or full soup cans, calisthenics such as chin-ups, push-ups, and sit-ups, or arm and leg extensions with exercise bands.

Just doing a few simple ten- to fifteen-minute strength-training routines at home or at the gym, two times a week, can turn the tide on muscle loss and activate your metabolism. You may notice an increase in the strength and the size of the exercised muscles in just a few weeks.

Strengthening exercises should be done at high intensity for the duration of the workout. For upper-body exercises, choose hand weights that make you work for the last two repetitions of any ten- to fifteen-rep set. If you're breezing through your sets, increase the weight, not the repetitions. For lower-body exercises done without weights, increase the repetitions to keep it challenging.

Here is a ten-minute strengthening workout you can do almost anywhere. Aim to do the workout every other day. For each exercise, perform two sets of ten to fifteen repetitions, resting for thirty seconds between sets.

Minutes 1 to 2: Biceps curl. Stand straight, arms at your sides, hands facing in toward your body, gripping weights. Slowly curl the weights up to your shoulders, turning your arms so that your hands face your chest. Slowly lower your arms to the starting position.

Minutes 3 to 4: Upper-arm presses. Stand straight, arms bent at the elbow, palms facing forward away from your body, gripping a weight in each hand. Slowly lift the weights straight up above your head, palms still facing out. Slowly lower the weights back to shoulder level.

Minutes 5 to 6: Upper body. While sitting on the edge of a chair, hold your back straight and put your feet flat on the floor. Balance hand weights on the tops of your legs, palms facing down, and arms bent. Slowly raise your bent elbows to shoulder height. Hold for two seconds, palms facing down. Slowly lower elbows back to your sides.

Minutes 7 to 8: Lower body. While sitting on the edge of a chair, hold your back straight and put your feet flat on the floor. Clasp your arms across your chest. Inhale and rise slowly out of the chair, keeping your back straight and your arms crossed so that you use only your buttocks and thighs. Slowly lower yourself back into the chair.

Minute 9: Abdomen. Sit on the edge of a chair and lower your torso so that your shoulders touch the back of the chair. Extend your legs, knees slightly bent, right ankle crossed over left. Lower your left heel to the floor. Grasping the sides of the chair, inhale and slowly raise your legs until they are parallel to the floor, using only your abdominal muscles. Do not strain your arms or neck. Hold for three seconds. Exhale and slowly lower your feet to the floor. After completing a set, repeat with left ankle crossed over right.

Minute 10: Back track. Stand in a slight lunge position — right foot back and straight, heel on floor, left foot forward, knee slightly bent. With your arms at your sides, exhale and slowly move your arms straight out toward your knee, then lift over your head. Bend your left knee as much as you can, without bending your right leg or lifting your right foot off the floor. Inhale as you slowly reverse the move, returning to your starting position. After completing a set, switch leg positions and repeat.

Weight training increases:	Weight training reduces:	Weight training improves:
muscle strength	body fat	balance
muscle mass	risk of diabetes	digestion
the body's average calorie-burning rate	risk of osteoporosis	mood
tendon and ligament strength	risk of heart disease	sleep
bone density	risk of colon cancer	
HDL cholesterol	lower back pain	
	arthritis pain	
	blood pressure	
	LDL cholesterol	

STRETCH!

Daily stretching is the best way to improve flexibility, one of the components of midlife fitness. The more flexible your body is, the better it can meet the demands of life and resist injury. You can find stretch classes at most fitness clubs, or you can learn stretching techniques from a variety of books and videos.

Here is a ten-minute stretching session. Aim to do the stretches every other day—when you wake up in the morning, after exercise, when you come home from work, or before you go to bed. Your body will thank you! For each exercise, hold the stretch for thirty seconds. Rest for fifteen to thirty seconds between each repetition. Breathe deeply while doing them.

Flexibility exercises should stretch your muscles, not strain them. If you feel sharp pain, stop.

Minutes 1 to 3. Lie on your back, knees bent, feet flat on the floor. Slowly lift your torso, keeping your head, shoulders, and feet on the floor. Hold for thirty seconds. Slowly lower your body to the floor. Repeat three times. Then, bend forward from a sitting position to stretch and relieve tension in the lower back. Hold for forty-five seconds, then put your hands on your thighs to help push your body back to an upright position.

Minutes 4 to 6. Stand with feet straight, arms at your sides, knees slightly bent. Inhale deeply. Exhale while slowly bending your body at the waist. Let your head hang loose as your fingers reach for the floor. Hold for thirty seconds. Slowly roll back up. Inhale. Repeat three times.

Minutes 7 to 10. Interlace your fingers, then straighten your arms out in front of you, palms facing out. Hold the stretch for a few seconds; repeat it. Then, interlace your fingers and turn palms upward above your head as you straighten your arms. Hold for ten seconds, rest, and repeat. Next, hold your right arm just above the elbow with your left hand. Now gently pull your elbow toward your left shoulder while looking over your right shoulder. Hold for ten seconds. Repeat using the opposite arm and hand and looking over your left shoulder.

PUTTING IT ALL TOGETHER: GET F.I.T.T. IN MIDLIFE

Consider this your exercise guide to be F.I.T.T.

Frequency. Once you've settled into a routine of exercise, do four to six aerobic workouts a week, and try to do one or more "long" workouts (over sixty minutes) per week. Exercising *less* will definitely produce benefit, but not enough. I try to do something every day to neutralize the ever-present stress in my life. Do two to three strength and conditioning workouts each week, and at least two times of stretching.

Intensity. Stay within the "feel-good zone," which means exercising fast enough to stimulate your mind and body but not so fast that you feel out of breath, gasping, or stressed. Make your effort as easy as possible so that you're able to exercise continuously for forty-five to sixty minutes without strain. Exercise should not hurt, but it should get your heart pumping. If possible, use a heart rate monitor, which is good for keeping you "in the zone."

Type. Do whatever type of exercise you enjoy (or could enjoy), can do regularly, and gives you the workout you need.

Time. Exercise forty-five to sixty minutes, at a time of day when you feel good and your schedule allows routine to be built. Choose a time of day that best suits your schedule. Is it early morning? This is a great choice to beat schedule surprises later in the day. Research has shown that those who begin exercising in the morning are more likely to be at it a year later. Another reason to set the alarm for morning exercise: After a night's fast, two-thirds of the calories you burn come from stored fat, which means a better "leaning" result coming from your workout.

If you do exercise first thing, grab a glass of energy-boosting juice first (4–6 ounces of apple, white grape, or unsweetened cranberry juice is great), then eat breakfast right after your workout. If you choose midday as your exercise time, don't let it interfere with your lunch time fueling or let the exercise break turn your lunch break into a frenzied spin. If you don't have at least an hour to invest, exercise will best be done at another time of day.

Your best move to combine lunch and a workout is to be sure you have your mid-morning power snack about two hours before your midday workout, then have a piece of fruit (a quicker release carbohydrate) and a twelve-ounce glass of water right before you warm up. Exercise for thirty minutes, freshen up, and then have at least a fifteen-minute lunch.

Is early evening best for you? Although this is a difficult time to stay consistent (easy to "just say no" after a hectic day!), it's a tremendous time to take advantage of exercise's stress-busting, energizing power. By diverting from your day's activities, you can downshift from stress to relaxation. It's a good time to review the day's events—the good, the bad, and the ugly—and get a pulse on how you feel about the events that occurred.

If you exercise after dinner, make it a half hour afterward so you won't be doing battle with your natural digestion process. Also, guard against exercising within half an hour of bedtime; your geared-up metabolism can interfere with restful sleep.

If you exercise outside, pay attention to the weather. If you live in a hot climate, be sure you are drinking lots and lots of water to replenish the fluids you are losing to perspiration. And don't forget your water needs even when it's cold outside. You can still exercise in the midst of winter, just be sure to bundle up in layered clothing that can "wick" the perspiration away from your skin. Be sure to cover your head and hands.

Whenever and wherever you exercise, use it as a time to stretch your spirit as well. It's a tremendous time to reflect, to pray, and to thank God.

REMEMBER THE PAYOFF

Eating well in our thirties, forties, fifties, and beyond is less about being thin and more about giving us energy to step into our busy days and strengthening our immune system. The same is true for exercise: The size of your waist is less of a payoff than the relaxed and exhilarated feeling you have after a brisk walk on a beautiful day.

As you are establishing your new fitness routine, keep your focus on how good you'll feel after you exercise. Keep envisioning exercise as a sword that cuts away at the stress response. Remind yourself of the long-term benefits you are getting: better energy, a better body, and better health. Choosing to exercise daily is giving a precious gift to yourself. Your body was created to reward you with feeling better quickly. Trust me, you will!

HORMONE BALANCING
ACTION STEPS: WEEK ELEVEN

Embrace a well-rounded workout—strength training, cardiovascular, and stretching—as your new way in midlife.

- ✔ *Continue to choose foods for your power meals and snacks that provide for stable blood chemistries.* Continue to record these in your Food-Feelings-and-Findings Journal. Review your diary for food choices, timing, and balance. Are there times in your day or entire days that reflect your enhanced feelings of well-being?

- ✔ *Be sure that you go into your exercise times well-fueled and hydrated.* Drink sixteen ounces of water right before you begin and six to eight ounces more every twenty minutes. Record the total quantity of water you are drinking each day.

- ✔ *Experiment with the power snack ideas on page 165 and break out of your rut!* Select at least three different snacks you intend to try this week. Be sure to add the necessary ingredients to your shopping list.

- ✔ *Check your heartbeat while walking.* Pick up the pace or intensity to bring your heart rate into your target zone—and keep it there. Continue walking at least five days a week.

- ✔ *Add five minutes of stretching into your day, at whatever time you can and will.* Use the stretching exercise suggestions on page 258.

- ✔ *Make an appointment with a personal trainer.* This is especially necessary if you are feeling insecure about adding weights into your workout or are just procrastinating. Even doing so just once will get you a personal routine and instruction.

✔ *Body-spirit balance step.* Exercise an "attitude of gratitude." As a woman in midlife, I have come to place high value on the power of giving thanks and rejoicing in all things. There is both spiritual and scientific wisdom behind gratefulness. It is imperative to our energy and well-being that we be thankful for what we have. Make a list of all the positive things and people God has placed in your life, including your own special giftings. Are you kind? Artistic? Good in business? Do you make people laugh? Read your list to yourself each night as you prepare for bed, adding to it as new thoughts arise. And let your bedtime prayer be that of "Thanks."

> *He gives strength to the weary*
> *and increases the power of the weak . . .*
> *those who hope in the LORD*
> *will renew their strength.*
>
> Isaiah 40:29, 31

LIGHT UP YOUR LIFE
AND LIFT YOUR MOOD

It's not just fluctuating hormones that bring on classic perimeno-pausal drops in serotonin; light deprivation can contribute as well. The more time you spend in low light conditions, the more likely you will feel tired and moody, eat too much, gain weight, and feel drowsy during the day—key symptoms of hormonal imbalance. Even if your hormones are not yet widely fluctuating, light deprivation can make you feel as though they are.

Until modern times, women got all the benefits of bright light simply by going about their normal routines. But today we have to consciously seek out the sun. Surveys show that most of us spend twenty-three hours a day indoors. As soon as we leave our home in the morning, we duck into a car, bus, or train. When we arrive at work, we scurry inside. After work, we run a few errands and then hurry back home. We spend most of our evenings cocooning indoors—reading, watching TV, catching up on paperwork, or being "mouse potatoes" (logging in massive time on our computers!). As a result, we get just a fraction of the light our bodies require. Surveys show that women get less light than men do.

LET THERE BE LIGHT!

We have all been created to thrive in sunlight. It's the spark of life without which there would be no plant growth, no photosynthesis, and no oxygen. It's all part of the Master's plan. God's first act of creation was to bring light to the darkness.

On a physical level, light causes normal physiological fluctuations that can affect the way we feel, think, and sleep. When we are getting adequate exposure to light, we produce adequate serotonin. But depending on personal sensitivity and the extent of light changes, if we get inadequate light, the effects can range from mild fatigue to severe depression.

Our brain's neurotransmitters respond well to sunlight. That's why we feel oppressed and trapped in urban centers or enclosed spaces. The more oxygen we get, the more alert we feel. And the more sunlight we get, the more feel-good chemicals the brain produces.

Sunlight is made up of a full spectrum of wavelengths or colors, each of which have an effect on your body. The full-spectrum wavelengths produced by the sun create feelings of emotional well-being and physical energy. A few minutes by a sunny window will brighten your day, and a walk outdoors can give you a tremendous boost! Even in the midst of winter when you can't see the sun, your body responds.

Most people underestimate the difference in light levels between indoors and out. Surprisingly, there is as much as 1,000 times more light available to us once we step outside. Sunlight, even on cloudy days, helps to set your biological clock, lifts your mood, strengthens your immune system, and produces vitamin D to keep you healthy and your bones strong.

Though not a replacement for natural sunlight, one type of artificial light helps you maintain proper energy levels and good spirits: warm incandescent light. Cool fluorescents have been shown to depress a person and deplete energy reserves. Different light—such as an increase and improvement in office lighting—has been found to result in decreased sickness and increased productivity.

ARE YOU SAD?

If you are desperately in need of light, you may be suffering from Seasonal Affective Disorder and may need full-spectrum bulbs that more closely simulate natural sunlight. This form of depression has been linked to inadequate exposure to light and may be caused by an improper balance of melatonin in the brain.

The symptoms of SAD are:

- a noticeable lack of energy
- a fairly constant level of sadness
- a desire to sleep as much as possible, but the sleep is fitful
- feeling listless and less creative than usual
- having less control of your appetite, resulting in significant weight gain

SAD needs to be treated appropriately. The best treatment results have been seen from the use of bright artificial light. Full-spectrum lights are now readily available for both home and commercial use.

LIGHT UP YOUR HORMONES!

There are three ways that bright light can help to relieve hormonal imbalance.

1. When sunlight falls on your bare skin, your body produces more vitamin D, a vitamin with proven mood-elevating properties and bone-protecting effects.
2. When light enters your eyes, it triggers the production of a variety of feel-good chemicals, serotonin included. This in turn lifts your spirits, suppresses your appetite, and helps boost your metabolism.
3. Bright light increases blood flow to your brain (which is somewhat limited as a result of dwindling estrogen), which in turn has a lifting action on depression and helps your memory and concentration. Studies have also confirmed that brightening your environment boosts physical energy and helps you sleep better at night.

HOW TO LIGHT UP YOUR LIFE

Here are some tips to let the sun shine in.

- Go for outdoor walks five or more times a week or find some other way to get twenty minutes of very bright light—1,000 lux or more—each day. (Lux is a way to gauge the intensity of light; 1,000 lux is the amount you'd get from about ten desk lamps.)

- Look straight ahead rather than down at the ground when you walk. A level gaze can more than double the amount of light that enters your eyes.
- Wear only lightly tinted sunglasses to block ultraviolet light but let in all the mood-boosting visible light.
- Open the blinds or curtains while you're home.
- Rearrange your furniture to face the windows.
- Install the brightest full spectrum lightbulbs your lamps will safely allow—even for your office desk lamp.
- Choose window seats on public transportation whenever possible.
- Plan a winter vacation in a sunny location. Just daydreaming about it will boost serotonin!

GETTING INTO THE PROPER RHYTHM

What keeps us tied to the light is a cleverly balanced internal clock, known as circadian rhythm, which synchronizes a wide variety of physiological systems including heart rate, body temperature, and, most importantly, sleep cycles. The clock is set by light; it can be reset by changes in the timing or duration of light exposure.

Most of us don't think twice about our circadian rhythms. We take for granted that we become tired and sleepy at night, awake and alert during the day. We notice the effects only if our internal clock is "out of sync"—when we gain or lose time or during seasonal changes in light. Even small changes can cause dramatic symptoms in some people. If you've ever experienced the lethargy, sleep disruption, difficulty concentrating, and general fuzziness that occur with jet lag, you know what I mean. Depending on the individual, those symptoms can persist for up to a week.

If you just want to smooth out your sleep-wake cycle and you don't have a serious circadian rhythm problem, try these simple measures to manipulate your exposure to light:

- If you have difficulty getting to sleep, turn off artificial lights for a half hour before your bedtime and use natural lighting, such as candlelight.

- If you get up in the middle of the night, avoid turning on bright lights. Light suppresses melatonin production and may make it more difficult to fall back to sleep. Put dimmer switches or night lights in bathrooms and hallways.
- If you have trouble getting up in the morning, maximize the amount of light in your bedroom as soon as you wake up. If you wake up too early in the morning, minimize the amount of dawn light. Wear a sleep mask or put blackout curtains on your windows. When you awake, keep lights dim to help gradually shift your usual pattern.
- Get plenty of sleep during the days and weeks before traveling across time zones, or when daylight-saving time begins (the first Sunday in April) and ends (the last Sunday in October). Starting fully rested will ease the transition.
- When traveling, get into the day/night cycle of the time zone you're going to as quickly as possible after you arrive. Don't hide in dark museums or hotel rooms upon arrival at your destination; stay out in the daylight.

THE LIGHT OF MY SOUL

Not only do we thrive in the light; we thrive when we lighten up! We get stressed and sick when we try to do too much or when we take ourselves too seriously. We can lighten our load when we come to understand that, although we don't always get to choose our circumstances, we do have a choice in how we respond to them—as victims or victors.

I believe the world has been given an abundance of peace, joy, and love by our Creator. When I don't see those things in my everyday life, I must ask what is blocking my light. Have my problems become my priorities? Are the obstacles in life all I can see?

A friend of mine calls obstacles "those ugly things that you see when you take your eyes off where you are going." My vision becomes distorted when I look at life only in terms of my expectations, others' standards, or what I myself can control. I believe that spiritually I have been given an incredible gift—spiritual eyes to see with 20/20 vision. When I can view my world through the eyes of my Creator, it makes all the difference in the way I live life. I am living in the Light.

HORMONAL BALANCING
ACTION STEPS: WEEK TWELVE

Get into the light!

✔ *Go outdoors five or more times a week*—walking, bike-riding, gardening, or the like. Find some way to get twenty minutes of bright light each day.

✔ *Continue to walk.* Increase the time to forty-five minutes, five times a week. Check your heart rate, and if you are not reaching your target zone for boosting your metabolism (see formula on page 253), pick up the pace and consider cross-training, adding in some new activities. If you are doing another form of aerobic exercise, monitor your heart rate to stay in the target zone.

✔ *Continue to choose foods for your power meals and snacks that provide for stable blood chemistries.* Review your diary for food choices that may contribute to better mood stabilization ("mood foods" on pages 97–98). Are there power foods that you do not normally choose? Plan to include each of these foods in at least one meal or snack this week. You might begin with broccoli or salmon. If you are not a fish eater, pick up some flaxseed.

✔ *Body-spirit balance step.* Lighten up—and *laugh!* There is extreme healing power that comes through laughter; it's the way we were designed. Laughter is one of the only activities other than exercise that produces stress-busting endorphins; it's a mini-workout! If life isn't striking you particularly funny right now, rent a comedy DVD or video (there are some great "blooper" compilations that are hilarious!), take the time to watch them, and just laugh. Call a funny friend; read some humorous books. I guarantee that something positive will happen in your emotions and spirit.

She can laugh at the days to come . . . .
Many women do noble things,
but you surpass them all.

Proverbs 31:25, 29

❄

CONGRATULATIONS!

You are now completing the action steps of the Hormone Balancing Plan. Consult the journal page you kept the very first week. Look at your answers to the questions on page 135 and answer them anew — *now.* What kind of progress have you made? What improvements in your symptoms? Review your initial goals; where are you in the process of achieving them?

Testing the results of different options can take some time. To be honest, I find that the waiting part is the hardest part. Maybe you are like me: Any time I make changes, I want to see immediate results — in a week or so, tops — and if that doesn't happen, I'm tempted to throw out that option and try another. Resist that temptation; you are on the right track.

Evaluate the lifestyle changes you have made so far and think about how many of them you wish to make permanent. Set new goals to work toward and choose a date to review them again in three months. Again, when making a change of any kind, most of us don't plan to fail. Instead, we fail to plan. Yet, planning is vital for healthy living to be a reality in our frenzied, frazzled lives. Plan to live well!

Receive my congratulations for completing this portion of your journey. You have learned much and are no doubt reaping the benefits. What will keep you on the road to your destination of hormone balance is continually putting into action what you have learned.

Part 4

SURVIVAL TIPS
TO MEN
ABOUT
THEIR WOMEN

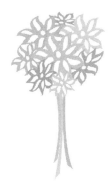

IF MAMA AIN'T
HAPPY...

From the moment we were separated in fifth grade to go watch "the movie," boys and girls have always wondered about the mystery of what they saw, what they know, and what they are experiencing.

That mystery continues for boys as they overhear often cryptic girl conversations about their "friend" coming to visit and as jokes about PMS abound. The subtle message from the adult men is often, "Women—you can't live with them, and you can't live without them." Or, "when hormones are raging, don't mess with them; it's like negotiating with a terrorist." Or, again, "if Mama ain't happy, ain't *nobody* happy!"

Times have changed; the wonder—and the confusion—hasn't.

When a woman's hormones go haywire, the men in the war zone can certainly get caught in the not-so-friendly fire. As *your* woman deals with the symptoms of hormones gone mad, let me encourage you to not get mad, and don't get her mad either.

Just the fact that you are reading this little chapter in this book says that your princess is making the choice to make the healthy difference in her life—to take charge of her hormones and well-being. She's probably been searching for some answers awhile, and the advice has been pouring in. Eat this. Don't drink that. Don't take hormones. Do. Nap. Relax. Exercise. Learn about soy and flax-seed.

But what about you? Here you are—the prince—and no one is asking you for or giving you a bit of advice. Yet, you are caught in the winds of change yourself, and may be dealing with some of your own version of hormone change. Questions abound: Will she make it through? Will *we*? Is this what life is going to be like from now on?

The problem is, you don't have all the physical changes of your own body to obsess on, so you have nothing to get your mind off the worries — and a good game of golf doesn't count. It's hard to go public with your concerns and fears because, well, it just doesn't seem like a "guy thing." And don't be surprised if your woman is so involved with her own emotions, thoughts, and worries that she has less time or interest in you or how you might be coping. Don't be surprised if your feelings come out "sideways," and you find yourself feeling a lot of the same physical symptoms as your wife. Cravings, weight gain, mood swings, insomnia — who knows, maybe even a hot flash or two!

For this reason, let me encourage you to get involved and knowledgeable about what your wife is going through. And stay involved. Ask questions, and read books like this one. As a matter of fact, now that you have this book in your hand, continue reading — right along with her. The healthy lifestyle principles employed to nurture your wife into hormonal balance and well-being can become the framework for your own healthy life and a healthier relationship. Encourage your wife to talk about her concerns and feelings, and painful as it is, talk about yours.

Most important, here is some lifesaving advice on how to be an absolutely perfect support in your vital role in times such as this:

1. Every day, find a way to mention how wonderful your wife looks, that you never realized how captivating a woman in midlife is, and that women who are twenty-something now seem shallow, immature, and well . . . boring.

2. Rave about the exciting and healthy ways you are eating together — and how much you love exercising together. Let her know how much you enjoy edamame as a snack instead of potato chips, and if you find her eating ice cream with fudge sauce at night, don't dare mention the fat and carb grams she counted off to you the night before.

3. Be a wellspring of empathy. Listen to all your wife's complaints about her body and show your undivided interest. Tell her you can't possibly know just how she's feeling, but you care.

4. Leave the camera at home when you go to the beach. If you see an unplanned photo of her before she sees it, destroy it.

5. If (or when) the grouchies overtake your wife, be amazed that she stays in such a great mood most of the time. Who wouldn't be a little cranky with all the changes she's going through, and with so little sleep. Never, never compare her current "edginess" now to her past experiences with PMS or a pit-bull.

6. Insist that she take a nap while you cook and clean the house, or pay someone to clean while you go get takeout.

7. Read books on foot massage and talk about how enjoyable it is to give a foot massage to her.

8. Realize that the most precious gift you can ever give to your wife is to make her *feel* loved.

9. Do not under any circumstances ever let the words "heavy," "weight gain," "thick-around-the-middle," or "sagging breasts" be used in your conversations.

10. Rejoice at the electric bills when they come, knowing that the air conditioner set on 68 is a small price to pay for her comfort. Joyfully invest in a heavy robe and fur-lined slippers—for the summer months.

Helpful Tips for Wives

- Generally, men really do care about their relationships with their wives. Be understanding and don't put all men in the same closet as the "clod" stereotype.

- Work with men as if they care. Give them a chance and learn to listen; you may have to break the ice.

- Try to understand what they are going through too. Communicate.

- Men may be going through midlife changes. They also may need air time or time to be alone.

- If you're married, why not ask your husband to pray with you?

Finally, a few tips to get you started:

- Accept what's happening. Don't go into denial.
- Menopause isn't an illness. It's demeaning to treat your wife as if she has a disease.
- Gain a little understanding of what makes hormones go haywire, and remember that every woman is different.
- Open the lines of communication. Listen without trying to fix.
- With awareness, you can respond rather than react, and you can make intelligent decisions.

Most of all, laugh together. It is, indeed, the best medicine.

Part 5

CONNECTING
THROUGH
CHANGE

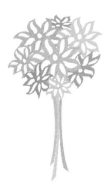

THE POWER FOR CHANGE

There is a time for everything,
and a season for every activity under heaven:
a time to be born and a time to die,
a time to plant and time to uproot . . .
a time to tear down and a time to build,
a time to weep and a time to laugh,
a time to mourn and a time to dance,
a time to scatter stones and a time to gather them,
a time to embrace and a time to refrain . . .
a time to keep and a time to throw away . . .
a time to be silent and a time to speak . . .
He has made everything beautiful in its time. He has also set eternity in the hearts of men; yet they cannot fathom what God has done from beginning to end.

Ecclesiastes 3:1–8, 11

Every transition begins with an ending. We have to let go of the old before we can embrace the new, both in our hands and our hearts.

CHANGES

It's ironic that the old catchword for menopause was "the change." As a woman in midlife, you can embrace this need for change. Your reproductive system, body composition, moods, skin, hair, libido, life roles, and relationships—everything is in transition, so rejoice in it!

Change is not new to us. Actually, in life nothing is more certain than change. In midlife, this is especially true. One minute we are young women, the next we are women in the middle, looking back to where we've been and looking forward to the rest of our lives.

As already mentioned (many times now!), midlife has a lot in common with puberty. Here we are, poised at the brink of second puberty, and we are once again concerned with changing bodies, changing roles, and changing views to how the world sees us and how we want to present ourselves to the world. We are preoccupied with hormonal ups and downs, and we are wondering what in the world we're going to do with our lives.

The changes of midlife are many.

Menstruation ends. Whether you see no more periods as a blessing or curse, the sudden loss of the monthly rhythm of life can cause disorientation. The reality that you can no longer reproduce life can become a deafening void of power, especially if you have not yet had children but hoped to.

Roles change. At the very time you are experiencing hormonal change, you may also be experiencing empty nest, and your role of mothering changes dramatically. You are forever "Mom," but as you see your children launching into their adult lives, the degree of input you once had takes a major shift.

Career changes. If you have been a full-time mother, you may decide to reenter the job market or go back to school. If you have worked outside the home all of your life to this point, you may consider retiring, changing jobs, or exploring a new career. With all the world turmoil, the decision may be made *for* you — through corporate downsizing.

Body changes. You spent twenty years growing up to being a young woman, and then twenty more years as a young woman. Now that image is changing. You certainly don't want to spend the next twenty years growing into an old woman, and then another twenty years being one. Yet your body tells you that this may be the unavoidable path. It's a disconcerting feeling, leaving us questioning if we are even the same persons we once were.

Relationships change. Friendship changes, children leaving, breakups, divorces, illness, deaths — whether part of the sweeping changes of this transition or the inevitable parts of life — all can bring a sense of loss and grief. Your parents are getting older, maybe ill, and you may find yourself facing decisions for their care, adding to your stress and a sense of life as being unfair.

Awareness changes. A greater awareness of missed opportunities commonly brings regrets in this stage of midlife. You become clearly aware of the sacrifices you've made for the life you have; you realize that some of your dreams may be forever unfulfilled.

Whatever your life experience, most every woman has to give up some dream of what she thought her life would be like. When that realization hits, it can be quite sobering and may require a time to process that pain, a time to grieve—letting go of what was in order to receive something new.

NEW LIFE

In any change, there is a golden opportunity to create new life. In this time of "the" change, we can see new life being created *in ourselves.* We become freer to choose where to direct our efforts and energies. Personal passions and interests burst forth, which many women funnel into new businesses, ministries, careers, volunteerism, or hobbies.

Women who do not fear this make a relatively smooth transition, emotionally and physically. Women who don't look at self as the original four-letter word learn how to balance their own needs with the needs and approval of others.

However, during times of confusion, we often draw inward. We pull back to sort things out, think things through, and reconcile old feelings. It is so easy to become isolated during times of such intense change, and it's not hard to find a wall to hide behind when you feel anxious or stressed. Many of us have become experts at building a "too busy" barrier to the support we most need—too busy to pay attention, too hurt to try, or too afraid to reveal our true selves to others, to God, or even to our own selves.

If you feel like this, live in it—just a bit—and enjoy the cocoon of reflection. It's one of the very important reasons not to miss the "body-spirit balance step" of the Hormone Balancing Plan. The time of midlife transition can become a perfect opportunity for personal renewal, for clicking into new connections with ourselves, and for deepening our spiritual lives, emerging as stronger, more authentic individuals. The changes within throw open doors to our emotions and souls that may have been shut tight for many years. It is not surprising that you may long for time alone, for a refuge that provides peace, quiet, and freedom from distractions and demands.

But also recognize that our wanting to be alone can lead to a hibernation of sorts and can immobilize us with an artificial sense that "no one but *me* is experiencing such turmoil and upheaval." It can be lifesaving to reach out and connect with other women who are experiencing the same sorts of changes you are. Finding emotional support on this rocky road of midlife can be a calming force. Getting counseling, joining or forming a support group, growing spiritually, and finding time to be with God and others can give you just the strength you need at a time you need it most.

CONNECTING WITH OTHERS: RELATIONAL BALANCE

Women holding onto one another for strength is a deeply resonant chord in this time of change. It is a truth vital to our emotional *and* physical well-being. You may find perspective and inspiration by listening to the wisdom of an older woman who has gone through this transition, asking her what it was like for her and what she learned. It can help to simply talk to someone who has been through menopause and has grown better and stronger from the journey. Spending time with someone who has already gone down the road you are now on can bring great comfort and learning. Or getting a group of women together who are in the trenches together can be enlightening and freeing. You don't have to reinvent every wheel.

Reach and Touch

Reach in — through reflection and journaling

Reach up — through prayer and worship

Reach out — through banding and bonding in small groups or friendships

We help each other by sharing our experiences, resources, and solutions for issues. We give a shoulder to lean on or cry on — and a buddy to chuckle with. It helps to laugh with other women that are right in the middle of the same experience — and might have found a new chin hair that morning too.

Speaking of such, Caron Loveless (my forever friend and inspiring author) reflected on the subject of midlife realities after she discovered an overnight sprouting of chin hair that she says was "the size of Mount Washington." In her sage wisdom, she was able to connect the horror of her discovery to her anxiety about this chapter of life, capturing something in me that instantly made me "feel better" and more connected to the sisterhood of women experiencing the same things I am. Forget a small Ya-Ya connection — this is big stuff:

> Renegade hair, like other midlife experiences, are good for exposing our private anxieties. They confirm one of our worst fears, that our bodies are beginning to have a mind of their own. No longer can we fully count on them to be there for us.
>
> These days I am standing in the foyer of midlife watching the door to what was closed behind me, and part of me, if I'm honest, sometimes feels cheated. Even though I've been given so much and still have a ways to go yet, it's easy for me to act like the child who gets a dollar bill from her daddy every day for a week, and then pitches a fit the next week when all he can give is fifty cents.
>
> If I'm going to make the most of these new, foreign experiences, if I'm going to get some good mileage out of them, I've got to find ways to translate them into a language my soul understands. It's easy to look in the mirror and obsess about the changing face of my life. But even more challenging is getting still enough to understand what God is trying to say to me through it.
>
> If I let them, even the smallest of midlife issues can bring a new level of clarity. They can help me sort through what's important, now . . .
>
> OK, so I missed the memo on chin hair.
>
> Now that it has shown up for the party, I plan to put it to work. I want it to be like a sign to me. I want it to say that the evidence is clear; there is no time to waste on lesser things. As I look in the mirror each morning, I'd like it to cause me to think, "Be fully here for your husband today . . . be fully alive to your sons . . . show up for your life today."

You can read more of Caron's reflections in *Honey, They Shrunk My Hormones* (Howard, 2003). Like everything she writes, her insights from the "trenches of midlife" move me to smile, nod—usually cry—and always feel slightly more sane and hungry for God's best. A personal favorite of mine is Caron's call to "embrace the wow of now—rejoice in all of its fresh, sweet and juicy possibilities."

Women connecting together is a time-honored practice. Whether it's an occasional get-together for tea, participating in a monthly meeting to discuss books or stocks, walking together in beautiful places, cooking and sharing a special meal, scrapbooking together, or coming together for prayer or baking bread, you will come away from these gatherings replenished and a bit more carefree.

Rather than accepting a fate of being forty, fat, miserable, flighty, and tired, we can hold onto each other for support, reclaiming our strength, vitality, and enthusiasm for life.

We are social beings who need regular contact with others to produce and perform optimally. Connecting with friends, especially those in whom we can confide and be natural, has been shown to promote mental health as well as physical well-being.

A Duke University study of nearly 1,400 people with heart disease revealed that those with even one good friend were three times less likely to die of a heart attack. Many studies have shown that people who have an array of social contacts seem to be more energetic and even get fewer colds than their less social counterparts. The simple truth is that friendship is good medicine!

Forming a Connection Group

Form a group of six to eight women. You do not have to be good friends or see each other outside the group. You do need to have a common interest, which may be nothing more than desiring to embrace the best of midlife or refusing to take on the worst.

Meet once or twice a month at someone's home or at a quiet cafe. Schedule about two hours for the meeting.

Allow time at the beginning for a check-in around the table or room for a quick update on how and what each person is doing. I suggest setting a time limit of five minutes per person; they can choose to fill the full five or choose not to.

Have one person be responsible for launching into a preselected topic: a book, a cultural issue, a challenge that is easily identifiable by the group. This woman will share for about five minutes and then open up for group discussion.

End promptly and announce the next meeting time.

The deeper truth is that replenishing relationships are those that help to get us well and keep us well. The energy and healing brought into your life by friends who appreciate who you are and who are there for you when you need them are precious and vital. This kind of friend challenges us to be our best and not to settle for staying stuck. They provide a new lens through which to look at our lives and ourselves.

HEALED — WELL AND WHOLE

Earlier, I told the story about the battle my daughters had over their stuffed donkey, Eeyore, and the sad result for his body as it was torn apart at the seams. That incident, and my seemingly continual identification of being pulled apart at the seams by conflicting demands, brings me to a reading that I find particularly empowering. It's a New Testament passage that is filled with hope and promise. It's a familiar story to many—a story about a woman with an "issue of blood":

> A woman who had suffered a condition of hemorrhaging for twelve years—a long succession of physicians had treated her, and treated her badly, taking all her money and leaving her worse off than before—had heard about Jesus. She slipped in from behind and touched his robe. She was thinking to herself, "If I can put a finger on his robe, I can get well." The moment she did it, the flow of blood dried up. She could feel the change, and knew her plague was over and done with . . .
>
> Jesus said to her, "Daughter, you took a risk of faith, and now you're healed and whole. Live well, live blessed!"
>
> Mark 5:27–28, 34 The Message

It certainly does take a risk of faith to step outside of what we are presently doing to do something different. Yet, we tend to do so only when the misery of where we are is greater than the fear of change. And as we take the first step, we receive the power to take that risk.

This is a woman who was at her wit's end—literally feeling as though she was bleeding to death, also being ripped apart at the seams. But she was drawn to the one who could bring wholeness back to her life. She was drawn to the one who she believed would be able to see clearly what she needed. We can imagine that he knew immediately of her loneliness and isolation from years of her illness, the frustration and hopelessness she felt after spending all she had on cures and treatments with no success. Her spirit as well as her body was crying out to be healed. And that is what she received—healing, wholeness, wellness, and blessing.

Isn't wholeness what we really want in our frenzied and frazzled lives of fulfilling so many roles? We want to feel like *whole* women—complete, real, and purposeful. We want to be sewn back together and not continue to be fragmented and torn.

We cannot obtain that wholeness by working harder, taking pills or potions, or ordering something through an infomercial special. Deep in our souls we know that; what we've been doing just isn't working. I believe that we receive that wholeness when we reach out—like the woman above—in faith.

REACHING OUT IN FAITH

My grandmother raised a family of twelve (*twelve!*) children in the hills of Kentucky, in over four decades from 1922 through 1962. Easily accessible medical care was not available to them for the majority of those years. Treating sickness involved making the ill as comfortable as possible and praying to God for healing.

It is true that in today's world of modern medicine and medical science, we have many more solutions and medical interventions available to us. Yet there are many within the health care systems who readily accept the powerful role that faith and prayer must play in modern-day medical miracles. Even health care professionals who don't personally have a relationship with God or believe in his power nonetheless acknowledge that people of faith often have unexplainable turnarounds in their health.

My grandmother taught me to "take care of what's

Friends for Life!

New research indicates that those who value love and friendship have higher levels of immunities and more of the other important body chemicals that keep us energized and strong. Just the memory of having loved or having felt loved can boost these power chemicals in your body, releasing peace-giving endorphins and serotonin.

yours"—that is, what's mine to control, such as my daily choices and my own body. She also taught me well to reach out in faith for the needs that are not mine to fill.

For me, reaching out in faith means that I open my hands to God and let go of what I am tightly holding onto, relinquishing the belief that I can control my world. Choosing to let go, to reach out and be rescued by God, is my path to living a life with spiritual connection. It nourishes my soul the same way that food and water nourish my body. Coming to my Creator with a genuine willingness to receive what he has planned for me, with faith that he loves me beyond measure, is the single most important step I can take to receive wholeness and peace.

When you reach out, even if it's just with a finger—a thimbleful—of faith, your new action brings healing, strength, and energy. Something powerful happens that is beyond the natural. May it be so for you—for life.

Live well, live blessed!

Part 6

RECIPES FOR HORMONE BALANCING

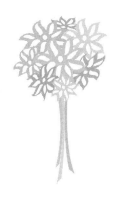

RECIPES FOR
HORMONE BALANCE

My take on healthy cooking and dining is guided by the premise that good health and good food are synonymous. It's an approach to food preparation and presentation that serves up meals that delight and nourish. This kind of cooking makes eating what we like the same as eating what is good for us. The food is fresh and flavorful, relying on herbs, garlic, fresh vegetables, fruits, and small amounts of high quality olive oil. There are no rich sauces, heavy starches, or fats to dull the senses.

Cooking and eating good food are great life pleasures. There's nothing wrong with that, except that for too long, "good" has meant "unhealthy" and was sure to be loaded with excess fats, sugars, and salt. "Healthy," by contrast, has been construed to be bland, boring, and tasteless. However, contrary to what many people have experienced, healthy food can—and should—be colorful, delicious, and quick and easy to prepare. For food to be enjoyable it needs to taste great; if it doesn't taste good, it has limited power to satisfy.

Each dish you'll find in the pages ahead is created from seasonally fresh and wholesome foods that are high in nutrients. The meals are designed to be naturally low in fat, calories, and sodium but high on flavor and beauty. And one more thing: They are designed for those of us who don't have the time (or often the energy) to plan and cook a meal after a busy day.

Let's face it: Time is short. We are often mentally and emotionally exhausted from the thousand and one demands of living life in this twenty-first century. On weeknights especially, spending less time in the kitchen becomes a clear necessity if we are to spend more time enjoying our family, friends, and hobbies. Too often in our catch-as-catch-can way of doing things, something is compromised: taste, health, or the entire satisfaction and fulfillment of making and enjoying a home-cooked meal.

With that said, I also believe that a major part of healthy living is not to spend any unnecessary time in the kitchen! My theory about cooking has always been, "If it takes longer to cook it than to eat it, *forget it!*" How about you?

I employ these basic pointers to "Make It Quick!" You might try them too.

Tip 1

Keep your pantry, fridge, and freezer well stocked with the basic ingredients for quick and easy food preparation. I'll give you a few tips below. Keep an ongoing grocery list and jot down items as soon as you begin to run low. If you wait until you are completely out of an item, it could cost you an unplanned trip to the store.

As flavorful, simple, and inexpensive as making your own stocks, sauces, and even salads can be, there are healthy, time-saving ingredients in your grocery store that can put convenience at your hand's reach.

Chicken stocks. Try Swanson Natural Goodness low-sodium, fat-free chicken broth; it's really "chickeny," without any aftertaste.

Canned beans. Try Goya or Eden Organic. The azuki beans and the soybeans, as well as all the usual black and white ones, are tasty and quick. Just rinse and drain in a colander and proceed as if they were just cooked.

Frozen, cooked shrimp. Already peeled and deveined, having a bag of these in the freezer is as handy as having a can of tuna in the pantry.

Fruit juices. One hundred percent pure juices (look for "no sugar added") are on your grocer's shelves and close to the dairy cases. They make wonderful marinades, bringing out the flavor of foods such as poultry and seafood. You can also buy frozen juice concentrates and use them as natural sweeteners to replace refined sugar.

Packaged, washed, and prepped salad packs and fresh vegetables. Now that producers are bagging shredded carrots, broccoli florets, cauliflower, and prewashed lettuces, there's no time excuse for not eating your veggies and salads. Yes, they cost more than whole heads of lettuce and bags of whole carrots, but you'll eat a lot more of it this way! The salads are ready to eat, and the vegetables work wonders for quick stir-fries and fresh vegetable platters.

Pasta sauce. Try Classico or Barillo. Of all the jarred sauces, these nongoopy, not-too-sweet, just-the-right-garlic formulas are ideal. They are made from naturally fresh ingredients with less than two grams of fat per serving.

Preshredded, 2 percent milk cheddar or mozzarella cheese. The convenience of grated hard cheeses (like Parmesan) isn't worth the compromise in flavor, but buying bags of preshredded, semi-soft cheeses makes sense. Store brands work just as well as Kraft or Sargento; just look for part-skimmed milk or 2 percent fat cheese.

Tomato salsas. These fat-free toppings or dips can be purchased fresh or jarred.

Tony Chachere's Creole seasoning. This adds a sassy surprise to your favorite recipes; find its green can in the spice aisle.

Tip 2

Since half the battle is just deciding what to prepare, pick out the meal you are going to try one or two days in advance and make sure you have the needed ingredients on hand. If you have a family, enlist them in this time of preparing—even assigning them the responsibility of a meal or two each week.

Tip 3

A recipe usually takes longer the first time you prepare it, so when you plan to make a new dish, give yourself the extra edge of time.

Tip 4

Keep a ready-to-cook kitchen. Do most of your food preparation on a countertop close to your sink. Declutter your countertops by storing your seldom-used appliances in less accessible cabinets. Use the drawer and cabinet closest to your cooking area to store knives, vegetable scrub brushes and peelers, stirring spoons, measuring spoons and cups, mixing bowls, colanders, cutting boards, scales, and graters. Keep your food processor and hand-held blender close so they are always handy for quick chopping, mincing, or blending.

Tip 5

Employ the professional kitchen technique called *mise en place*, which means organizing and pre-prepping your ingredients so that you are ready to cook. It does wonders for speeding your cooking time, keeping your sanity, and assuring a dish without forgotten ingredients.

Tip 6

Trim time by freezing food. One way to streamline your food preparation is to look for the recipes that can be doubled or tripled, then frozen for later use. Nothing can calm frenzied nerves after a busy day — overflowing into a busy night — like a meal that can be pulled out of the freezer and heated up in a jiffy!

If you're marinating and grilling two chicken breasts, why not do a dozen? Then you can freeze them individually in small plastic zip-top bags. Later they can be popped into the microwave for a quick chicken sandwich or salad. French Toast is simple and quick to make on order, but you can speed up the process even more by having pregrilled slices frozen and ready to pop in the toaster. When making it, I quadruple the recipe and use an entire loaf of bread, freezing the grilled toasts into individual bags. On early mornings, they can be popped out of the freezer and into the toaster for a quick but delicious breakfast.

The same goes for any number of dishes — from lasagna to meat loaf. I also use this theory when I'm picking up takeout. Rather than getting two healthy Chinese meals to bring home, I bring home four and freeze the two extras in small bags for quick meals. Combined with my own just-made brown rice, it makes a terrific mealtime treat weeks later.

CHOOSE WHERE TO BEGIN

Even if you're fired up with the ambition to cook healthy, great-tasting meals, you still have to consider how much time you have to shop and cook. Begin by taking stock of what you are doing now for breakfast, lunch, and dinner. Try tackling just one of the day's meals at a time. Which would you like to change first?

You might start with eating breakfast, perhaps for the first time since you were five years old. Or you may start packing a more interesting lunch—one that's healthier too. It may be one fabulous dinner a week or elements of health sprinkled throughout your life. What is important is getting started with the energy and excitement of a new way of eating!

Whatever you choose as your first step, the rewards of better eating come quickly: boosted energy and moods, superior concentration and alertness, a better memory—and putting a stop to hot flashes. Your Hormone Balancing Meal Plan on pages 171–73 is your road map to your new healthy destination.

ON-THE-GO BREAKFASTS

For breakfast, you might like to find some simple, everyday alternatives to cereal or a bagel—or the worst choice, no breakfast at all! Breakfast can be made in less than five minutes; even healthy homemade muffins can be made in advance and frozen for a quick pop-out. Mixing up a power shake in the blender before bed and holding it in the refrigerator makes a blender breakfast a breeze.

These are my favorite breakfasts because they can be put together with minimal fuss or effort—and in a jiffy.

Baked Breakfast Apple

1 small golden delicious apple, cored	¼ tsp. cinnamon
2 tbs. old-fashioned oats	½ cup nonfat ricotta cheese
1 tbs. raisins	½ cup apple juice

Place the apple in a microwaveable bowl. Mix together the oats, cinnamon, and raisins. Fill the cavity of the cored apple with the mixture. Pour the apple juice over the apple and cover it with plastic wrap. Microwave on high for 1 minute. Turn the dish around halfway and microwave for 1 minute more. Spoon the ricotta cheese onto a plate and top it with the apple and the heated juice mixture.

Makes 1 serving, giving 1 complex carbohydrate (oats), 2 oz. protein (ricotta), and 1 simple carbohydrate (apple, the juice, and the raisins).

Nutritional analysis per serving: 183 calories, 30 g carbohydrate, 14 g protein, 1 g fat (6% calories from fat), 100 mg sodium

Breakfast Shake

½ c. frozen fruit	¼ c. pasteurized egg whites or egg substitute*
1 c. skim or soy milk	2 tbs. ground flaxseed
1 tsp. vanilla	2 tbs. wheat germ
1 tsp. honey	2 tbs. wheat bran

Blend frozen fruit in blender. Try strawberries, mangoes, peaches, blueberries, and bananas. (Don't throw away your very ripe bananas; peel and freeze in freezer bags and use for your shakes.) Add remaining ingredients and continue blending till smooth.

Makes 1 serving, giving 1 complex carbohydrate (wheat germ and bran), 2 oz. protein (milk), and 1 simple carbohydrate (fruit).

*You may buy cartons of pasteurized egg whites in the dairy case. Or, you may make your own, "coddling" a whole egg by placing in boiling water for 30 seconds. Crack egg; use egg white immediately.

Nutritional analysis per serving: 200 calories, 32 g carbohydrate, 16 g protein, 2 g fat (10% calories from fat), 176 mg sodium

Ricotta Breakfast Sundae

½ banana, quartered lengthwise	¼ c. crushed pineapple, canned in own juice
½ c. nonfat ricotta or cottage cheese	2 tbs. Grape Nuts or low-fat granola
¼ c. strawberries sliced, or blueberries	1 tsp. honey or all fruit pourable syrup

Place the banana quarters star-fashioned on a small plate. Scoop ricotta cheese onto the center of the plate, just topping the points of the bananas. Surround with the other fruit; then sprinkle with cereal. Drizzle with honey or all fruit syrup.

Makes 1 serving, giving 1 complex carbohydrate (cereal), 2 oz. protein (ricotta), and 2 simple carbohydrates (fruit).

Nutritional analysis per serving: 224 calories, 42 g carbohydrates, 15 g protein, 1 g fat (4% calories from fat), 111 mg sodium

Toasted Cheese and Pears

2 slices whole wheat bread	1 tbs. raisins
½ pear, thinly sliced	2 oz. mozzarella or soy cheese

Top bread with pears and raisins. Place cheese on pear-raisin layer. Broil until cheese is bubbly.

Makes 1 serving, giving 2 complex carbohydrates (bread), 2 oz. protein (cheese), and 1 simple carbohydrate (apple and raisins).

Nutritional analysis per serving: 332 calories, 41 g carbohydrate, 19 g protein, 11 g fat (30% calories from fat), 586 mg sodium

Hot Oatcakes

4 egg whites	⅔ c. old-fashioned oats, uncooked
1 c. nonfat ricotta cheese	¼ tsp. salt
1 peeled banana	Nonstick cooking spray
1 tsp. vanilla	4 tbs. all fruit jam or pourable all fruit syrup

Measure the egg whites, ricotta, banana, vanilla, oats, and salt into a blender or food processor and blend for 5 to 6 seconds. Spoon 2 tbs. of the batter into a hot skillet sprayed with nonstick spray. Turn the oatcakes when bubbles appear on the surface; cook for 1 more minute.

For 1 serving, spread 3 oatcakes with 1 tbs. all fruit jam or syrup. Makes 12 three-inch oatcakes. Freeze the leftovers in individual freezer bags. When ready to use, toast the pancakes to thaw and heat.

Makes 4 servings, each giving 1 complex carbohydrate (oats), 2 oz. protein (ricotta and egg whites), 1 simple carbohydrate (jam), and 1 added fat.

Nutritional analysis per serving: 160 calories, 28 g carbohydrate, 12 g protein, 7 g fat (0% calories from fat), 97.5 mg sodium

Recipes for Hormone Balance

PART 6

Orange Vanilla French Toast

6 egg whites, lightly beaten	1 tsp. cinnamon
1 c. skim or soy milk	6 slices whole wheat bread
1 tsp. vanilla	All fruit preserves or mashed fresh fruit
½ c. orange juice*	

Beat together egg whites, milk, vanilla, orange juice, and cinnamon. Add bread slices one at a time, letting the bread absorb liquid in the process. May let the bread sit for a few minutes. Spray nonstick skillet with cooking spray, then heat. Gently lift the bread with spatula into skillet and cook until golden brown on each side. Serve topped with ½ c. fresh fruit or 1 tbs. (no sugar) all fruit preserves. You can freeze the extras and pop them in the toaster on a busy morning.

Makes 3 servings, giving 2 complex carbohydrates (bread), 2 oz. protein (eggs, milk), and 1 simple carbohydrate (juice and fruit).

* Add the juice of half a fresh orange, and it's even better!

Nutritional analysis per serving: 329 calories, 55 g carbohydrate, 20 g protein, 3 g fat (7% calories from fat), 529 mg sodium

Hot Apple-Cinnamon Oatmeal

⅔ c. old-fashioned oats	1 tbs. raisins
1 c. skim or soy milk	½ tsp. vanilla
½ c. unsweetened apple or white grape juice	½ tsp. cinnamon
	2 tbs. ground flaxseed

Bring milk, juice, and oats to a boil. Gently cook for 5 minutes, stirring occasionally. Add raisins, vanilla, cinnamon, and flaxseed; let sit covered for 2 to 3 minutes to thicken. This recipe also cooks well in the microwave — just combine first three ingredients in a microwavable bowl and cook for 3 to 4 minutes on high, then add remaining ingredients.

Makes 1 serving, giving 2 complex carbohydrates (oats), 2 oz. protein (milk), and 1 simple carbohydrate (juice and raisins).

Nutritional analysis per serving: 357 calories, 63 g carbohydrates, 17 g protein, 4 g fat (10% calories from fat), 131 mg sodium

Nut Butter Danish

2 slices 100% whole wheat bread	1 tbs. natural peanut butter or soy nut butter
½ banana	8 oz. skim or soy milk

Slice banana lengthwise and place with inside facing down on one slice of bread. Top with other slice of bread and nut butter. Broil until nut butter is slightly brown and bubbly. It's really delicious! Have with an 8-ounce glass of milk for added protein.

Makes 1 serving, giving 2 complex carbohydrates (bread), 2 oz. protein (nut butter and milk), and 1 simple carbohydrate (banana).

Nutritional analysis per serving: 374 calories, 53 g carbohydrates, 18 g protein, 10 g fat (25% calories from fat), 418 mg sodium

Huevos Rancheros

Nonstick cooking spray	¼ tsp. Creole seasoning, divided
One 10-inch whole wheat tortilla, fat free	1 tsp. Mrs. Dash seasoning, divided
¼ c. black beans, cooked and drained	2 egg whites or ½ c. egg substitute
¼ c. chicken stock	¼ c. tomato salsa

Spray tortilla with nonstick cooking spray. Place into heated nonstick skillet and grill until crisp. Set aside. Spray skillet again with cooking spray. Add black beans, chicken stock, 1/8 tsp. Creole seasoning, and ½ tsp. of Mrs. Dash; quickly sauté until beans are easily mashed. Spread on tortilla. Spray skillet with cooking spray again; add egg substitute and remaining seasonings. Scramble. Spoon on top of beans and top with salsa.

Makes 1 serving, giving 2 complex carbohydrates (tortilla, beans), 2 oz. protein (eggs, beans), and 1 simple carbohydrate (salsa).

Nutritional analysis per serving: 200 calories, 38 g carbohydrate, 14 g protein, 1 g fat (5% calories from fat, with egg substitute), 599 mg sodium

TERRIFIC LUNCHES

Lunches are a wonderful opportunity to brown bag a healthy meal as an alternative to fast food or ordering in. You can certainly get a "two-for-one" if you make extra at dinner the night before and lunch on healthy leftovers the next day, or save kitchen clean-up time by making tomorrow's lunch while making dinner.

Terrific Tuna Grill

1 can (6½ oz.) solid white tuna, water-packed, drained	2 tbs. orange juice
¼ c. carrots, shredded	1 tsp. Dijon-style mustard
½ stalk celery, diced	½ tsp. Creole seasoning
1 apple, diced (½ c.)	2 slices 100% whole wheat bread
2 tbs. light mayonnaise	1 plum tomato, sliced
2 tbs. plain, nonfat yogurt	Nonstick cooking spray

Combine the tuna, carrots, celery, and apple. In a separate bowl stir together the mayonnaise, orange juice, yogurt, mustard, and Creole seasoning until blended. Pour the mixture over the tuna, stirring to coat it. Divide the tuna mixture into two portions, spreading one portion onto one slice of bread (use or reserve the other portion for another sandwich). Top with tomato slices and the other slice of bread. Spray a nonstick skillet with nonstick cooking spray and heat on medium high. Grill the sandwich until brown.

Makes 4 servings, each giving 2 complex carbohydrates (bread), 3 oz. protein (tuna), and 1 simple carbohydrate (veggies and fruit).

Nutritional analysis per serving: 300 calories; 37 g carbohydrate, 28 g protein, 4.7 g fat (14% calories from fat), 38 mg cholesterol, 567 mg sodium

Hot Carrot-Cheese Melt

| 1 grated carrot (about ½ c.) | 2 slices whole wheat bread |
| 3 oz. grated mozzarella or soy cheese (about ¾ c.) | Tomato slices and lettuce leaves, if desired |

Mix together carrots and cheese. Spread bread with carrot-cheese mix. Grill in nonstick skillet till cheese melts. Add tomato slices and lettuce (and even alfalfa sprouts).

Makes 1 serving, giving 2 complex carbohydrates (bread), 3 oz. protein (cheese), and 1 simple carbohydrate (carrots).

Nutritional analysis per serving: 361 calories, 45 g carbohydrate, 25 g protein, 9 g fat (22% calories from fat), 578 mg sodium

Swiss Stuffed Potatoes

1 baking potato (about 5 oz.)	1 oz. (¼ c.) part skim mozzarella or soy cheese, shredded
¼ c. part skim or nonfat ricotta cheese	
¼ tsp. Creole seasoning, or salt and pepper to taste	Paprika

Preheat oven to 400 degrees. Wash the potato and dry. Microwave potato by pricking and cooking on high for 2 minutes, turning and microwaving for another 2 minutes, or until tender.

Once cooked, cut the potato in half lengthwise and scoop out most of the pulp, leaving ¼-inch shell. In a bowl, mash the potato pulp with the ricotta cheese and seasoning. Stir in the mozzarella cheese and spoon the mixture into the potato shells. Sprinkle with paprika.

Increase the oven temperature to broil; broil the stuffed potato shells for 3 to 5 minutes or until they are heated through and lightly browned on top.

Each serving gives 1 complex carbohydrate (potato), and 2 oz. protein (cheese).

Nutritional analysis per serving: 339 calories, 28 g carbohydrate, 17 g protein, 9 g fat (24% calories from fat), 513 mg sodium

Tempeh Sandwiches

Because of its solid, chewy texture, tempeh (which is made from soybeans and grains) is a good meat substitute; you can find it at your natural foods store.

2 medium garlic cloves, minced	3 tsp. olive oil
¼ tsp. kosher salt	4 large ½-inch thick slices of whole grain bread, halved crosswise
¼ c. light mayonnaise	
1 tbs. finely chopped fresh flat-leaf parsley	
One 8-oz. package of tempeh	4 ripe plum tomatoes, thinly sliced crosswise
2 tbs. balsamic vinegar	
½ tsp. Tony's Creole seasoning	Half a small bunch of arugula or baby spinach, stems trimmed
1 medium red onion, thinly sliced crosswise	

On a work surface, using the flat side of a large knife, crush the garlic with ¼ teaspoon salt until almost pureed. In a small bowl, stir together the garlic, mayonnaise, and parsley.

Using a thin sharp knife, cut the block of tempeh crosswise on an angle into 12 slices about ¼ inch thick. Brush the slices on both sides with the vinegar and season lightly with Tony's Creole seasoning (or salt and pepper).

In a large nonstick skillet, cook the onion in 1 teaspoon of the oil over moderate heat, stirring occasionally and separating the onion into rings, until slightly softened, about 5 minutes. Transfer the onion to a plate.

Add 2 remaining teaspoons of the oil to the skillet and swirl the pan to coat. Add the tempeh in a single layer and cook over moderate heat, pressing lightly with a spatula and turning once, until lightly browned, 1½ to 2 minutes per side.

Toast the bread and spread each piece with the prepared parsley-mayonnaise. Place the tempeh on 4 pieces of toast and top with the onion rings, tomatoes, and arugula. Sandwich together with the other pieces of toast and serve at once.

Makes 4 servings, each one giving 2 complex carbohydrates (bread, tempeh), 3 oz. protein (tempeh), and 1 simple carbohydrate (veggies).

Nutritional analysis per serving: 331 calories, 43 g carbohydrate, 24 g protein, 7 g fat (26% calories from fat), 585 mg sodium

Tofu Burritos

2 tsp. olive oil	⅓ c. chopped fresh cilantro
2 c. chopped bell peppers (preferably red, yellow, and green)	¼ tsp. Tony's Creole Seasoning
	Salt and pepper, to taste
One 14 oz. package soft tofu, drained, cut into cubes	Four 8-inch diameter whole wheat tortillas, fat free
2 large garlic cloves, chopped	Shredded romaine lettuce
2 tsp. chili powder	Tomato salsa
¼ c. chopped green onions	

Heat olive oil in a large nonstick skillet over medium-high heat. Add bell peppers and sauté until beginning to soften, about 2 minutes. Add tofu, garlic, green onions, and chili powder and sauté until bell peppers are soft, about 3 minutes. Mix in cilantro; season with Tony's Creole seasoning and, if desired, salt and pepper. Remove from heat. Wrap flour tortillas in plastic and warm on low in microwave. Arrange flour tortillas on work surface. Spoon ¼ of filling into center of each, top with shredded romaine and salsa. Fold tortilla sides over ends of filling; roll up to enclose filling. Cut each burrito in half, place on plate.

Makes 4 servings, each one giving 1 complex carbohydrate (tortilla), 2 oz. protein (tofu), and ½ simple carbohydrate (peppers, salsa).

Nutritional analysis per serving: 227 calories, 25 g carbohydrates, 16 g protein, 7 g fat (28% calories from fat), 394 mg sodium

Grilled Turkey and Cheese Sandwich

2 tsp. Dijon-style mustard	1 ripe plum tomato, sliced
2 slices 100% whole wheat bread	2 oz. skinned turkey breast, fully cooked and sliced
1 oz. or ¼ c. grated low-fat Swiss or soy cheese (such as Jarlsberg Lite or Veggie-Slices)	

Spread the mustard on each slice of bread. Put 2 tablespoons of cheese, the tomato, and the turkey on one slice of bread. Sprinkle with the additional cheese and top with the remaining slice of bread. Grill the sandwich on a hot griddle or a nonstick skillet coated with nonstick spray. Cook until the bread is lightly browned and the cheese melts. Serve with fresh fruit.

Makes 1 serving, giving 2 complex carbohydrates (bread), 3 oz. protein (turkey and cheese), and 1 simple carbohydrate (fruit).

Nutritional analysis per serving: 307 calories, 32 g carbohydrate; 29 g protein; 7 g fat (20.5% calories from fat), 551 mg sodium

Garden Gazpacho

A wonderful chilled soup that cools the summertime! Serve with a salad topped with black beans or grilled chicken.

1 red pepper	12 oz. tomato juice
1 green pepper	1 tbs. white wine vinegar
½ cucumber	1 tsp. Tabasco
2 tomatoes	¼ tsp. cumin
½ small red onion, chopped	1 tsp. Creole seasoning
2 garlic cloves, minced	¼ c. fresh basil or cilantro, chopped
12 oz. V – 8 juice	

Seed and dice peppers, cucumbers, and tomatoes; combine with remaining ingredients. Chill.

Makes 12 servings, ½ cup each, each giving ½ simple carbohydrate (soup).

Nutritional analysis per serving: 22 calories, 5 g carbohydrate, 1 g protein, 0 fat, 312 mg sodium

Eggless Egg Salad Sandwich

1 lb. firm tofu, drained	½ c. diced celery
½ c. diced red onion	¼ c. shredded carrot
½ tsp. garlic, minced	1 tbs. light mayonnaise
2 tsp. Dijon mustard	½ tsp. each kosher salt and cracked black pepper
8 (1-oz.) slices pumpernickel bread	
15 (⅛-inch thick) slices cucumber	
10 (⅛-inch thick) slices large tomato	
5 Bibb lettuce leaves	

Combine first 8 ingredients in a bowl; beat at medium speed of a mixer until combined (mixture will not be smooth). Spread ⅔ c. tofu mixture evenly over 1 bread slice; top with 3 cucumber slices, 1 lettuce leaf, 2 tomato slices, and 1 bread slice. Repeat procedure with remaining ingredients.

Makes 4 sandwiches, each giving 2 complex carbohydrates (bread), 3 oz. protein (tofu). and 1 simple carbohydrate (carrot and tomato).

Nutritional analysis per serving: 242 calories, 38 g carbohydrates, 14 g protein, 5.5 g fat (20% of calories from fat), 765 mg sodium

Chicken of the Land or Sea Apple Sandwich

¾ c. water-packed chicken or tuna	¼ tsp. Tony's Creole Seasoning, or salt and pepper to taste
1 small stalk of celery, chopped	2 tsp. Dijon mustard
1 small chopped apple	1 whole wheat pita, halved
1 tbs. reduced-calorie mayonnaise	Romaine lettuce leaves

Mix together first 6 ingredients. Stuff into 2 halves of pita lined with lettuce.

Makes 1 serving, giving 2 complex carbohydrates (pita), 3 oz. protein (tuna or chicken), and 1 simple carbohydrate (apple).

Nutritional analysis per serving: 332 calories, 40 g carbohydrate, 25 g protein, 8 g fat (22% calories from fat), 650 mg sodium

Grilled Tofu Salad

Sweet and spicy Asian seasonings flavor this composed salad.

Two 1-lb. blocks of firm tofu	1 tbs. black bean chili paste
2 medium garlic cloves, minced	4 c. arugula or baby spinach, tough stems removed
2 tbs. honey	
2 tbs. peanut oil	¾ c. Miso-Carrot Dressing (recipe follows)
2 tbs. soy sauce	

1. If you can't find firm tofu, you can use regular tofu as follows: Place the tofu blocks between two baking sheets and weigh down the top with two or three heavy cans. Let stand at room temperature for 30 minutes, occasionally pouring off the excess liquid. Proceed with the recipe.

2. Slice each tofu block ½ to ¾ inch thick and pat the slices dry.

3. In a small bowl, stir together the garlic, honey, peanut oil, soy sauce, and black bean chili paste. Spread half of the marinade in the bottom of a large nonreactive baking dish and top with the tofu slices. Spread the remaining marinade over the tofu, covering it completely. Let stand for 1 hour before grilling.

4. Preheat a stovetop grill or the broiler. If using a grill, spray with nonstick spray before heating. Grill or broil the tofu, turning once, until caramelized and brown, 2 to 3 minutes per side. Brush with any remaining marinade. Let cool. Cut each piece into wide strips if desired.

5. To serve, line plates or a platter with the arugula or spinach and set the tofu on top. Drizzle the Miso-Carrot Dressing on the salad.

Makes 6 servings, each giving 3 oz. protein (tofu) and 1 simple carbohydrate (carrots, veggies). Serve with brown rice or Seeded Tortilla Triangles (page 308) as complex carbohydrate.

Nutritional analysis per serving: 320 calories, 26 g protein, 17 g carbohydrate, 9 g fat (23% calories from fat), 920 mg sodium

Miso-Carrot Dressing

Use this hearty dressing for the tofu salad (preceding) or with broiled chicken or fish. Find miso at your natural foods store.

2 small carrots, coarsely chopped	1 tbs. rice wine vinegar
2 small garlic cloves, peeled	1 tbs. olive oil
One ¾-inch piece of fresh ginger	¼ tsp. sugar or honey
⅔ c. fresh carrot juice	2 tsp. minced fresh basil
2 tbs. yellow miso	2 tsp. minced fresh cilantro

In a blender, combine the carrots, garlic, ginger, carrot juice, miso, vinegar, olive oil, and sugar and blend until perfectly smooth. Transfer to a jar. Just before serving, stir in the basil and cilantro. Makes 1-¼ cups; the dressing can be refrigerated for up to 4 days.

Nutritional analysis for 2 tablespoons: 32 calories, 1 g protein, 4 g carbohydrate, fat 1.5 gm

POWER SNACKS

Simply Edamame

1-lb. bag frozen edamame	Coarse salt to taste

Fill a 5-quart kettle three-fourths full with water and bring to a boil. Have ready a bowl of ice and cold water. Cook frozen edamame in boiling water until bright green, 2 to 3 minutes, and transfer with a slotted spoon to ice water to stop cooking. Drain edamame well and trim stem ends of pods for easier eating. Edamame may be prepared 4 hours ahead and kept in a bowl, covered with a damp paper towel and plastic wrap, at cool room temperature.

Just before serving, toss edamame with salt to taste.

Seeded Tortilla Triangles

2 tbs. flax seeds	2 tbs. poppy seeds
2 tbs. sesame seeds	½ tsp. coarse kosher salt
2 (10- to 12-inch) whole wheat tortillas	2 tbs. Eggbeaters with 1 tbs. water

Preheat oven to 350°F. Stir together flax, sesame, poppy seeds, and kosher salt. Put 1 tortilla on each of 2 baking sheets and brush with some egg mixture. Sprinkle with seeds to coat, then cut each tortilla into long thin triangles with a sharp knife. Bake in upper and lower thirds of oven, switching position of sheets halfway through baking, until crisp and lightly golden, 15 to 20 minutes total. Transfer triangles to racks to cool. Repeat with remaining 2 tortillas. Makes 16 triangles; 8 triangles give one serving.

Chef's note: Triangles may be made 1 day ahead and kept in an airtight container at room temperature. If triangles lose crispness, recrisp in a 350°F oven about 5 minutes.

Roasted Red Pepper Dip

1 (7-oz.) bottle roasted red bell peppers, drained	2 garlic cloves, crushed
1 c. reduced-fat firm silken tofu (about 6 oz.)	1 (16-oz.) can cannellini beans or other white beans, rinsed and drained
⅓ c. fresh parsley leaves	1 tsp. minced seeded jalapeno pepper, may add more for extra spice
2 tbs. lime juice	
1 tbs. extra-virgin olive oil	
¼ tsp. kosher salt	Sliced jalapeno pepper (optional)
½ tsp. Tony's Creole seasoning	
½ tsp. ground cumin	

Chop roasted peppers to measure ¼ c.; set aside. Place remaining roasted peppers, tofu, and the next 8 ingredients (tofu through beans) in a food processor, and process until smooth. Spoon mixture into a bowl; stir in reserved ¼ c. bell peppers and minced jalapeno. Cover and chill. Garnish with a sliced jalapeno, if desired. Makes 2½ cups (serving size: ⅓ cup).

Lowfat Hummus

Lovers of hummus will appreciate this reduced-fat version.

1 tbs. cumin seeds	⅓ c. fresh lemon juice, or to taste
19-oz. can chickpeas (about 2 c.), drained	
12 oz. low-fat silken tofu	2 tbs. extra-virgin olive oil, or chili oil
4 cloves garlic (roasted, if desired)	¼ c. chopped fresh flat-leafed parsley leaves plus additional for garnish
1 tsp. Tony's Creole seasoning	
Kosher salt and cracked black pepper, to taste	

In a dry small heavy skillet, toast cumin seeds over moderate heat, shaking pan, until seeds are a shade darker, and transfer to a plate to cool. Rinse and drain chickpeas. Drain tofu. In a food processor purée chickpeas, tofu, garlic, cumin seeds, Creole seasoning, lemon juice, and 1 tablespoon oil until chickpeas are smooth. Stir in parsley and salt and pepper to taste. Drizzle dip with remaining tablespoon oil and garnish with parsley. Serve dip with pita toasts and/or crudités.

Makes about 3 cups; ⅓ cup is one serving.

Fresh Fruit Tofutti Shake

A wonderful snack or breakfast!

1 banana	4 oz. vanilla yogurt
¼ c. crushed unsweetened pineapple, canned	1 c. peaches or strawberries, frozen
¼ c. orange juice	2 tbs. ground flaxseed
8 oz. silken tofu	

Combine all ingredients in blender. Mix well. Makes 2 servings.

If preparing more dinners is your goal, you certainly don't need to plan and shop for seven full menus each week. Factor in meals out and the meals you might have in the freezer, or those quick meals when evening schedules don't allow a leisurely sit-down dinner with the family or friends. If you've been doing very little home cooking and have a realistic goal of making one or two dinners a week, perhaps you can cook on the weekend when you have the time.

Seared Shrimp with Edamame, Corn, and Tomato Saute

A colorful and delicious side dish reminiscent of succotash.

1 lb. shrimp, peeled, deveined, and marinated in white wine Worcestershire sauce	2 c. shelled cooked edamame beans (from about 26 oz. of pods)
1 tsp. olive oil	One 14½-oz. can diced tomatoes in juice
½ c. finely chopped red onion	
4 garlic cloves, minced	1 c. corn
1¾ tsp. ground cumin	½ c. canned chicken broth
½ tsp. Tony's Creole seasoning	2 tbs. chopped fresh basil
Salt and pepper, to taste	

Marinate shrimp for 15 minutes to one hour.

Heat oil in large nonstick skillet over high heat. Add onion and garlic; sauté until golden, about 5 minutes. Add shrimp; cook 2 to 3 minutes and remove. Add cumin and Creole seasoning; stir 1 minute. Add tomatoes with their juices; bring to boil. Reduce heat to medium or medium-high and cook until most liquid has cooked away, about 5 minutes. Stir in edamame, corn, and broth. Simmer until most broth is absorbed, about 6 minutes. Add shrimp. Season with salt and pepper. Transfer to bowl. Sprinkle with basil and serve.

Makes 4 servings, each giving 1 complex carbohydrate (corn, edamame), 2 oz. protein (shrimp, edamame), and 1 simple carbohydrate (tomatoes).

Nutritional analysis per serving: 227 calories, 28 g carbohydrate, 22 g protein, 3 g fat (12% calories from fat), 733 mg sodium

16 oz. soy tempeh or 3-grain tempeh, cut into ½-inch pieces	12 oz. broccoli, stems peeled and cut into ½-inch pieces, florets cut into 1-inch pieces
¼ c. light soy sauce	
2 tbs. rice vinegar	2 tbs. water
3 garlic cloves, minced	1 tsp. honey
2 tsp. minced peeled fresh ginger	1 tsp. cornstarch
	1 tsp. olive oil
⅛ tsp. dried crushed red pepper	½ c. chopped red bell pepper
	¼ c. edamame, shelled
¼ c. green onion, chopped	

Stir together soy sauce, vinegar, garlic, ginger, and crushed red pepper in medium bowl to blend. Add tempeh and let it marinate 1 hour at room temperature.

Steam broccoli until crisp-tender, about 3 minutes. Set aside.

Strain marinade from tempeh into small bowl; set tempeh aside. Whisk 2 tablespoons water, honey, and cornstarch into marinade. Heat oil in large nonstick skillet over high heat. Add marinated tempeh, bell pepper, and edamame and sauté 4 minutes. Add broccoli and marinade mixture and sauté until broccoli is heated through and sauce thickens, about 3 minutes. Transfer to bowl. Sprinkle with green onion and serve.

Makes 4 servings, each giving 1 complex carbohydrate (tempeh), 2 oz. protein (tempeh), and 1 simple carbohydrate (broccoli, peppers).

Nutritional analysis per serving: 250 calories, 23 g carbohydrate, 20 g protein, 7 g fat (26% calories from fat), 585 mg sodium

Chili Con Tofu

Spicy chili seasonings work wonders for the bland flavor of tofu. For a more substantial, spicy chili, use the same weight of tempeh in place of the tofu. Since tempeh is not packed in water, there is no need to pat it dry before sautéing, but stir in up to one extra cup of water in Step 4 when adding the beans.

2 tbs. olive oil	1 tsp. ground cumin
1 medium red onion, finely chopped	35-oz. can of Italian peeled tomatoes in juice
4 medium garlic cloves, minced	1 c. canned tomato sauce
	½ tsp. dried oregano
2 large poblano chiles, seeded and finely chopped	1 tsp. salt
	1-lb. block of extra-firm tofu, drained and patted dry
1 large red bell pepper, seeded and finely chopped	19-oz. can of black beans, drained
1 medium jalapeño chile, minced	½ c. finely chopped fresh cilantro
⅓ c. pure chili powder	

This chili is best if it stands for at least 1 hour or overnight.

1. In a large, heavy, nonreactive casserole dish, heat 1 tablespoon of the oil. Stir in the onions, garlic, poblanos, bell pepper, and jalapeño and cook over moderate heat, stirring occasionally, until slightly softened but not browned, about 10 minutes. Add ¼ c. of the chili powder and the cumin and sauté another minute.

2. Coarsely chop the tomatoes and add them to the casserole with their juice and the tomato sauce. Stir in the oregano and salt and bring to a simmer over moderate heat. Reduce the heat to moderately low and simmer, stirring occasionally, until all the vegetables are soft, about 15 minutes.

3. Meanwhile cut the tofu into ½-inch dice and pat dry. Place in a bowl and toss with the remaining 4 teaspoons chili powder. In a large nonstick skillet, heat the remaining 1 tablespoon oil. Add the tofu and cook over moderately high heat for 3 minutes to lightly toast the chili powder. Season with ¼ teaspoon salt. Transfer the tofu to the casserole. Add ⅓ c. of water to the skillet and scrape the bottom of the pan with a wooden spoon to loosen the browned bits. Add the liquid from the skillet to the casserole.

4. Stir the black beans into the chili and simmer, stirring frequently, until the flavors are blended, about 10 minutes. Before serving, stir half of the cilantro into the chili; sprinkle the rest on top.

Makes 6 servings, each giving ½ complex carbohydrate (beans), 2 oz. protein (beans, tofu), and 1 simple carbohydrate (tomatoes).

Nutritional analysis per serving: 276 calories, 39 g carbohydrate, 16 g protein, 6 g fat (21% calories from fat), 485 mg sodium

Herb Crusted Grouper

4 grouper fillets (5 oz. each)	2 tbs. chopped fresh herbs (cilantro, basil, rosemary, and thyme)
¼ c. white wine Worcestershire sauce	
1 tsp. Creole seasoning	¼ c. Dijon mustard
½ c. dried bread crumbs (purchased)	1 tbs. olive oil

Preheat oven to 375° F.

Marinate grouper in Worcestershire sauce for at least 15 minutes or up to 1 hour. Season fish with seasoning and roll in bread crumbs and herbs. Spread mustard on top of fish and roll in bread crumbs once more. Spray a nonstick skillet with cooking spray; add olive oil and heat. Sear fish in hot skillet on both sides, then transfer to oven and roast until done and browned.

Makes four servings, each giving ½ complex carbohydrates (bread crumbs), 3 oz. protein (fish).

Nutritional analysis per serving: 142 calories, 7 g carbohydrate, 24 g protein, 2 g fat (13% calories from fat), 623 mg sodium

Brown Rice Pilaf

1 tsp. olive oil	1¾ c. chicken stock
½ red onion, diced	½ tsp. Creole seasoning
2 cloves garlic, minced	2 c. instant brown rice
1 tbs. chopped fresh herbs (cilantro, basil, rosemary, and thyme)	

Spray a medium saucepan with cooking spray; add olive oil and heat. Add diced onion and garlic, and lightly sauté about 1 to 2 minutes; then add chicken stock, seasoning, and herbs. Let mixture come to a boil, then stir in brown rice. Let boil for 1 minute, turn down heat to low and cover. Let simmer for 5 minutes, uncover skillet, and fluff rice with fork. Cover again. Let sit for another 5 minutes.

Makes 6 servings, each giving 1 complex carbohydrate.

Nutritional analysis per serving: 106 calories, 19 g carbohydrate, 2.5 g protein, less than 1 g fat (9% calories from fat), 136 mg sodium

Tuscan Broccoli

1 tsp. olive oil	½ tsp. Creole seasoning
2 cloves garlic, minced	1 tsp. Mrs. Dash seasoning
2 tbs. capers, rinsed	1 bunch (1-¼ lb.) broccoli, cut into florets and trimmed of tough stalks
1 tbs. chopped fresh rosemary (or 1 tsp. dried)	
½ c. chicken stock (fat-free/low salt)	

Spray a large nonstick skillet with cooking spray. Add olive oil and heat over medium heat. Add garlic, capers, seasonings, and rosemary; sauté until the garlic is golden, about 30 seconds. Add the broccoli florets and chicken stock. Reduce heat and cook covered until broccoli is crisp tender and cooking liquid is reduced, about 5 to 7 minutes. Ladle into serving dish, tossing together.

Makes 4 servings, each giving 1 simple carbohydrate.

Nutritional analysis per serving: 57 calories, 8 g carbohydrate, 4 g protein, 1 g fat, (16% calories from fat), 688 mg sodium

Firm tofu keeps its shape during cooking, so it's the best choice for stir-fry. On its own, it's rather mild, but once added to the dish, tofu acts as a sponge, absorbing the savory flavors of the sauce.

1½ lbs. asparagus	¾ c. chicken stock, or canned low-sodium chicken broth
2 tsp. cornstarch	
1 tbs. water	3 tbs. tamari or soy sauce
2 tbs. canola oil	5 tsp. rice wine vinegar
4 cloves garlic, minced	¾ tsp. Asian sesame oil
1 large onion, chopped	¾ tsp. salt
1 lb. shiitake mushrooms, stems removed and caps sliced, (or white mushrooms, sliced)	2 lbs. firm tofu, cut into 1½-inch cubes
	3 c. brown rice, cooked
1 tbs. toasted sesame seeds (optional)	

1. Snap off the tough ends of the asparagus and discard them. Cut the asparagus into 1-inch lengths. In a large pot of boiling, salted water, or in microwave, cook the asparagus for 3 minutes. Drain and set aside.

2. In a small bowl, combine the cornstarch and water; set aside

3. In a wok or large frying pan, heat the oil over moderately high heat. Add the garlic. Stir-fry until fragrant, about 30 seconds. Add the onion and stir-fry until softened, about 3 minutes. Add the sliced mushrooms and stir-fry until brown, about 5 minutes.

4. Stir in the stock, tamari or soy sauce, 3 teaspoons of the vinegar, the sesame oil, and the salt. Simmer for 2 minutes. Stir the cornstarch mixture from step two, add it to the pan, and simmer until the sauce has thickened. Add the tofu and simmer for 3 minutes. Add the asparagus from step one and simmer until hot, about 2 minutes longer. Stir in the remaining 2 teaspoons vinegar. Serve over ½ cup brown rice, topped with the sesame seeds, if desired.

Makes 6 servings, each giving 1 complex carbohydrate (½ c. brown rice), 2 oz. protein (tofu), and 1 simple carbohydrate (asparagus, mushrooms).

Nutritional analysis per serving: 261 calories, 27 g carbohydrate, 18 g protein, 9 g fat (30% calories from fat), 875 mg sodium

RECIPES FOR HORMONE BALANCING

Chicken Pad Thai

1 lb. boneless, skinless chicken breasts (about 3), cut into 1-inch cubes	¾ lb. linguine
	3 tbs. canola oil
	4 cloves garlic, chopped
6 tbs. Asian fish sauce	2 c. broccoli florets
½ lb. firm tofu, cut into ¼-inch cubes	1 red bell pepper, cut into pieces
1 c. water	⅔ c. salted peanuts, chopped fine
2 tbs. lime juice	
1½ tsp. rice-wine vinegar	2 c. bean sprouts
3½ tbs. sugar or honey	½ c. lightly packed cilantro leaves
¾ tsp. salt	
¼ tsp. cayenne	Soy sauce or tamari, if desired

1. In a small bowl, combine the chicken and ½ tablespoon of the fish sauce. In another bowl, combine the tofu with another ½ tablespoon of the fish sauce. In a medium glass or stainless steel bowl, combine the remaining 5 tablespoons fish sauce with the water, 1½ tablespoons of the lime juice, the vinegar, sugar, salt, and cayenne.

2. In a pot of boiling, salted water, cook the linguine until done, about 12 minutes. Drain.

3. Meanwhile, in a wok or large frying pan, heat 1 tablespoon of the oil over moderately high heat. Add the chicken and cook, stirring, until just done, 3 to 4 minutes. Remove. Put another tablespoon of oil in the pan. Add the tofu and cook, stirring, for 2 minutes. Remove. Put the remaining 1 tablespoon oil in the pan, add the garlic, bell pepper, broccoli, and cook, stirring, for about 2 minutes or until tender.

4. Add the pasta and the fish-sauce mixture. Cook, stirring, until nearly all the liquid is absorbed, about 3 minutes. Stir in the chicken, tofu, and ⅓ c. peanuts. Remove from heat. Stir in the remaining ½ tablespoon lime juice, the bean sprouts, and half the cilantro. Top with the remaining peanuts and cilantro. May add soy sauce to top of each plate for added flavor.

Makes 6 servings, each giving 2 complex carbohydrates (pasta), 4 oz. protein (chicken, tofu), 1 simple carbohydrate (broccoli), and 1 added fat.

Nutritional analysis per serving: 381 calories, 42 g carbohydrate, 33 g protein, 9 g fat (19% calories from fat), 875 mg sodium

BBQ Grilled Tempeh Sandwiches

⅓ c. ketchup	1 (8 oz.) package tempeh
1 tbs. brown sugar	1 red bell pepper, cut in half
1½ tsp. olive oil	1 yellow bell pepper, cut in half
1½ tsp. cider vinegar	
1 tsp. Dijon mustard	1 red onion, cut into ½-inch thick slices
¼ tsp. chili powder	
¼ tsp. low-sodium soy sauce	Cooking spray
¼ tsp. hot sauce	4 (1½ oz.) whole wheat hamburger buns
1 garlic clove, minced	

Prepare grill. Combine the first nine ingredients in a small bowl, stirring with a whisk. Cut tempeh in half lengthwise; cut slices in half. Brush tempeh slices, bell peppers, and onion with the ketchup mixture. Place on grill rack coated with cooking spray; grill 4 minutes on each side or until the tempeh is thoroughly heated. Remove the tempeh, bell peppers, and onion from grill. Cut bell peppers into ½-inch wide strips; separate onions into rings.

Place 1 tempeh slice on bottom half of each bun. Top each tempeh slice with one-fourth of bell peppers, one-fourth of onion, and top half of bun.

Makes 4 servings, each giving 2 complex carbohydrates (bun), 2 oz. protein (tempeh), and 1 simple carbohydrate (veggies).

Nutritional analysis per serving: 309 calories, 42 g carbohydrates, 19 g protein, 8.5 g fat (12% calories from fat), 530 mg sodium

Garlic Spinach

2 tsp. extra virgin olive oil	1 lb. baby spinach, prewashed
4 cloves of garlic, minced	Red pepper flakes (optional)
½ tsp. Creole seasoning	Lemon, half

Spray a shallow roasting pan with cooking spray. Add garlic and olive oil, sauté about one minute until garlic begins to foam. Add seasoning and spinach; sauté lightly until spinach begins to wilt. Add red pepper flakes to taste, if desired. Squeeze lemon juice over spinach, toss again, and serve immediately.

Makes 4 servings, each giving 1 simple carbohydrate.

Nutritional analysis per serving: 248 calories, 21 g carbohydrate, 23 g protein, 8 g fat (29% calories from fat), 349 mg sodium

Chopped Tomato Salad

2 medium ripe tomatoes, chopped	3 tbs. chopped fresh basil
	1 tbs. balsamic vinegar
1 medium red bell pepper, chopped	2 tsp. freshly squeezed lemon juice
1 medium yellow bell pepper, chopped	2 cloves garlic, minced
	1 tsp. dried oregano
1 small red onion, chopped	½ tsp. Creole seasoning
2 tsp. capers	Salt and freshly ground black pepper to taste

Mix together all ingredients in a large bowl; cover and refrigerate 1 hour. Equally divide and place a mound of salad on each serving plate.

Makes four servings, each giving 1 simple carbohydrate.

Nutritional analysis per serving: 32 calories, 7 g carbohydrate, 1 g protein, 0 g fat, 196 mg sodium

Black Bean, Corn, and Edamame Salsa

2 c. black beans, drained and rinsed	1 tbs. olive oil
1 c. frozen corn kernels, thawed	4 cloves garlic, minced
1 c. shelled, cooked edamame beans	Juice of two limes
2 plum tomatoes, diced	1 tbs. balsamic vinegar
½ red onion, minced	1 tsp. cumin
1 serrano pepper, minced	2 tsp. hot pepper sauce
1 tbs. chopped fresh cilantro	1 tsp. Creole seasoning

In a large bowl, combine all ingredients and mix well. Allow to marinate at least one hour before serving.

Makes ten ⅓ cup servings, each giving 1 complex carbohydrate (corn, beans) and 1 oz. protein (beans, edamame).

Nutritional analysis per serving: 106 calories, 15 g carbohydrate, 8 g protein, 1.5 g fat, 118 mg sodium

Too hot to turn on the oven? Try stovetop poaching; it's a moist and flavorful cooking technique and will help you to keep your cool.

1 c. white wine (or de-alcoholized wine or more chicken stock)	1 lb. of salmon, cut into four filets
2 c. chicken stock (fat free/low salt)	1 lb. asparagus, trimmed of tough stalks
1 whole shallot, quartered	2 c. Black Bean, Corn, and Edamame salsa (see previous recipe)
2 cloves garlic, minced	
2 sprigs fresh thyme	2 c. fresh spinach leaves, washed and stemmed
2 bay leaves	
¼ tsp. cracked black pepper	1 tbs. chopped chives
½ tsp. Creole seasoning	1 lemon, sliced

Add first eight ingredients to a large nonstick skillet to make poaching stock; bring to boil. Add salmon and asparagus spears; simmer 5 to 7 minutes until done. Spoon black bean and corn salsa onto plate. Add fresh spinach leaves and placed poached salmon and asparagus spears on top of the leaves. Sprinkle with chopped chives and garnish with twisted lemon slice.

Makes 4 servings, each giving 2 complex carbohydrates (corn, beans), 4 oz. protein (salmon, beans), and 1 simple carbohydrate (asparagus).

Nutritional analysis per serving: 316 calories, 38 g carbohydrate, 32 g protein, 4 g fat (11% calories from fat), 405 mg sodium

Snapper with Tomato and Feta Cheese

2 ripe tomatoes, sliced	1 tsp. dried basil
2 cloves garlic, finely minced	1 lemon, thinly sliced
1 lb. red snapper fillets* (½ inch thick — fresh preferred)	½ tsp. dried oregano
	⅓ c. feta cheese, crumbled

Arrange the tomato slices on the bottom of a 9-inch glass pie dish. Sprinkle the garlic over the tomatoes and arrange the fish over the top. Sprinkle the basil over the fish. Place the lemon slices on top; sprinkle with the oregano and the crumbled feta cheese. If possible, let the fish sit for about 30 minutes. Cover the fish with vented plastic wrap and microwave on high for 4½ to 5 minutes. Let it stand for 5 minutes before serving.

Makes 4 servings, each giving 3½ oz. protein (fish and feta) and ½ simple carbohydrate (tomato).

* May substitute tilapia, orange roughy, or any mild white fish

Nutritional analysis per serving: 190 calories, 7 g carbohydrate, 27 g protein, 6 g fat (28% calories from fat), 318 mg sodium

Herb-Roasted Potatoes

2 lbs. (about 5 large) red-skinned potatoes, scrubbed and quartered	1 tsp. Mrs. Dash seasoning
2 cloves garlic, minced	1 tbs. chopped fresh rosemary (or 1 tsp. dried)
2 tsp. olive oil	
½ tsp. Creole seasoning	

Preheat oven to 450° F. Spray a shallow roasting pan with cooking spray. Add potatoes, garlic, olive oil, seasonings, and rosemary; toss to coat potatoes. Spread in an even layer. Bake until the potatoes begin to brown, 20 to 30 minutes, turning them once midway through roasting.

Makes 6 servings, each giving 1 complex carbohydrate.

Nutritional analysis per serving: 93 calories, 18 g carbohydrate, 1.5 g protein, 1 g fat (10% calories from fat), 104 mg sodium

Spaghetti Pie

6 oz. vermicelli or whole wheat pasta	8 oz. can stewed tomatoes
	6 oz. can tomato paste
2 tsp. olive oil	¾ tsp. dried oregano
⅓ c. grated Parmesan cheese	¼ tsp. salt
2 egg whites, well beaten	½ tsp. garlic powder
½ lb. ground turkey	1 c. part-skim ricotta cheese
½ c. chopped onion	½ c. shredded mozzarella cheese
¼ c. chopped green pepper	

Cook pasta according to package; drain. Stir olive oil and Parmesan cheese into hot pasta. Add egg whites, stirring well. Spoon mixture into a 10-inch pie plate. Use a spoon to shape spaghetti into a pie shell. Microwave uncovered on high 3 minutes or until set. Put aside.

Crumble turkey in colander, stir in onion and green pepper. Cover with plastic wrap and microwave on high 5 to 6 minutes, stirring every 2 minutes or until no longer pink.

Let drain well. Put into a bowl and stir in tomatoes, tomato paste, and seasonings. Cover and microwave on high 3½ to 4 minutes, stirring once. Set aside.

Spread ricotta evenly over pie shell. Top with meat sauce. Cover with plastic wrap and microwave on high 6 to 6½ minutes; sprinkle with mozzarella cheese. Microwave uncovered on high 30 seconds, or until cheese melts.

Makes 6 servings, each giving 2 complex carbohydrates (pasta), 3 oz. protein (turkey, cheese), and ½ simple carbohydrate (tomatoes).

Nutritional analysis per serving: 248 calories, 21 g carbohydrate, 23 g protein, 8 g fat (29% calories from fat), 349 mg sodium

ONE LAST POINT TO REMEMBER

It's your day-to-day eating that counts most for health and wellness, not what you eat on your birthday or Thanksgiving Day. One day, or even a week, of less-than-great eating will not send your body headfirst into a hormonal hurricane; it just might feel like it! It's progress, not perfection, that counts.

Are you ready for your hormones to come into balance? Then get cooking and enjoy this new adventure of discovering wonderful new flavors, new tastes, and new recipes, all the while restoring hormonal balance and greater health. You will love the results as you begin to nourish your body and spirit now through menopause.

Glossary

Adrenal glands: two small glands, situated above each kidney, that produce a variety of hormones involved in immunity, sodium-potassium balance, sexuality, and the control of stress

Adrenaline: a chemical produced in the adrenal system on signal from the brain to put the body on alert for survival. Adrenaline surges in the stress response, heightening the alerting and protective systems in the body and stimulating the fight-or-flight reaction.

Artificial menopause: menopause brought on by surgery or chemotherapy

BeEst: dual natural estrogen, a chemical composition similar to what the body produces

Biophosphates: group of drugs that prevent bone loss and reduce the risk of fractures

Black cohosh: herb that suppresses LH and is a popular remedy for hot flashes

Blood sugar: the more correct term is blood glucose, but blood sugar is the popularized and more widely known. Blood sugar levels have a powerful influence on our health and well-being, affecting our energy, moods, concentration, appetite, and disease risk.

Carbohydrate: an essential nutrient that is a part of the foods we eat, mostly coming from plant foods. The energy it provides for vital body functions is critical to the human body, as are the essential vitamins, minerals, phytochemicals, and fibers it carries with it. Carbohydrates are a storage form of the sun's energy, occurring through the process of photosynthesis, and become 100 percent energy for our body.

Refined: complex carbohydrate (starch) that has been stripped of its fibers and most of its vitamins, minerals, and phytochemicals.

These carbohydrates break down quickly during digestion and are quickly released into the bloodstream to be metabolized.

Whole: carbohydrates in the least processed form — harvested grains, fruits or vegetables that have been prepared without destroying their nutritive value or fiber. These carbohydrates are broken down more slowly in digestion, gradually and steadily releasing glucose into the system to be burned.

Chemical gymnastics: wide fluctuations in body chemistries occurring when the body is overstimulated with overconsumption of food or stress (emotional or physical), or underprovided for with adequate fueling or sleep

Circadian rhythm: internal clock that is set by light and synchronizes various physiological systems such as heart rate and sleep cycles

Complementary medicine: using lifestyle as preventative medicine and making appropriate adjustments to stabilize the body processes

Complete proteins: those proteins that contain all eight essential amino acids; primarily found in foods of animal origin

Conditioning exercises: those exercises that tone, shape, and define muscles through repetitive movement against resistance

Cortisol: a hormone produced by the adrenal system in response to chronic stress that exerts great influence on immune function, blood pressure, pulse rate, metabolism, and fat storage. Cortisol inhibits the production of testosterone, the precursor to estrogen, and increases the production of insulin.

Diabetes: disease in which the hormone insulin is not present in sufficient amounts

Dopamine: a vital chemical neurotransmitter that brings high levels of energy but in an alert, aroused, "get-things-done" state. Abnormally high levels of dopamine result in high anxiety — to the point of aggressiveness and paranoia, and the brain alert stimulates production of hormones that contribute to the fat-cell lock down.

Edamame: young soybean pods

Endorphin: a "morphine-like" brain chemical that kills pain, reduces anxiety, and contributes to feelings of self-esteem, euphoria, and emotional well-being. Responsible for what is termed the "runner's high," endorphin is produced in the brain when you exercise and when you laugh. Endorphins are natural calming agents that release you from the stress response.

Epinephrine: one of two primary stress-response hormones, produced in the adrenal glands

ERT (estrogen replacement therapy): see HRT

Estradiol: hormone produced by fertile ovaries

Estriol: hormone produced from the conversion of estrone

Estrogen: key sexual hormone, produced primarily in the ovaries before menopause and in body fat after, that is responsible for the transition from childhood to womanhood; among other things, serves in the regulation of the menstrual cycle

Estrone: hormone produced from the conversion of estradiol in the fat cells

Fat: an essential nutrient that is part of the foods we eat — found in animal products and plant oils. It is vital for growth, lubrication, hormone production, and the absorption of certain vitamins. It is also a concentrated source of calories that are easily stored as fat on the body.

Fats that clog arteries include:

Saturated fat: Found in dairy and meat products, including milk, cheese, ice cream, beef, and pork. It also can be found in coconut and palm oils, nondairy creamers, and toppings.

Trans-fat: Formed when vegetable oils are hardened into solids, usually to protect against spoiling and to maintain flavor. Examples include stick margarine and shortening, deep-fried foods such as French fries and fried chicken, and pastries, cookies, doughnuts, and crackers. Read the ingredient list of any processed foods you buy. If you see the words "partially hydrogenated," look for a different product, especially if it is one of the first three ingredients. Hydrogenation is a manufacturing process that converts a polyunsaturated or monounsaturated oil into a saturated fat.

Fats that do not clog arteries include:

Monounsaturated fat: Found in olive, canola, and peanut oils. These fats increase good HDL cholesterol and decrease bad LDL cholesterol and thus the risk of disease.

Omega–3 fatty acids (EPA and DHA oils): Found in all fish and seafood, particularly cold-water fish such as salmon, albacore tuna, swordfish, sardines, mackerel, and hard shellfish. The only plant source is flaxseed. Omega–3 fatty acids decrease triglycerides and bad LDL cholesterol. They reduce the tendency of the blood to form clots, stabilize blood sugars, improve brain function, and reduce inflammation.

Polyunsaturated fats decrease both bad LDL and good HDL cholesterol, so they aren't the desired choice. These fats are those in corn oil, cottonseed oil, safflower oil, sesame oil, sunflower oil, as well as avocado, sunflower seed kernels, sesame seeds, almonds, walnuts, and pecans.

Fat storage formula: when stressed, a lack of self-care (sedentary lifestyle, sleep deprivation, erratic, or overeating) and states of imbalance (illness, hormone dysfunction, depression, or worry) put the body into a survival mode of energy storage through the slowing down of the metabolism

Fibrocystic disease: benign breast disease

F.I.T.T. – frequency, intensity, type, and time of exercises

FSH (follicle-stimulating hormone): a pituitary-stimulating hormone that travels to the ovary, stimulates ovarian eggs to produce estrogen, and stimulates an egg to be released at ovulation.

Flavonoids: antioxidant-like compounds found in fruits and vegetables. They are thought to be health-protective, potentially guarding against everything from cancer to heart disease.

Glucose: a simple sugar that is the building block of starch. In the small intestine, digestive enzymes break down large molecules of complex carbohydrates (starch) into smaller molecules. These and simple carbohydrates (sugars) are then broken into simpler monosaccharides (glucose, fructose, and galactose) to be absorbed into the bloodstream, where they are available as a source of energy to the cells. Glucose is the most critical of these monosaccharides, because it is the source of fuel used by the brain, central nervous system, and lungs. If your diet doesn't provide enough carbohydrate to supply glucose, the brain will signal a shortage, and muscle tissue will be broken down to supply the shortfall.

Glycemic index: a ranking from 0 to 100 that estimates the glucose-loading power of a food—whether a food will raise blood sugar levels dramatically and quickly (fast release), moderately (quick release), or just a little (slow release). Carbohydrate foods that break down quickly during digestion have the highest glycemic values—the blood sugar increases rapidly; carbohydrates that break down slowly, releasing glucose gradually into the bloodstream, have low glycemic ratings.

Glycogen: the body's readily available storage supply of glucose, stored in the liver and muscle. The body maintains a certain level of glucose in the blood to serve the brain, lungs, and central nervous system.

Hormone: a chemical messenger substance produced in the body that has a specific regulatory effect on the activity of certain cells or organs

Hormone Balancing Plan: a systematic, twelve-week plan to restore and maintain hormone balance

HRT (Hormone Replacement Therapy): prescription estrogen alone or in combination with the synthetic version of progesterone to counteract the effects of menopause

Hydrogenation: process in which vegetable oils are hardened into solids, producing trans-fatty acids

Hypertension: high blood pressure

Hyperthyroidism: condition in which the thyroid produces excess amounts of thyroxine, overstimulating organs and speeding up many of the body's functions

Hypothalamus: neural centers in the brain just above the pituitary gland that regulate fluid balance, sleep, blood sugars, and production of all hormones

Hypothyroidism: underactive thyroid gland that can result in weight gain, heavy menstrual bleeding, fatigue, dry skin, painful joints, and mood swings

Insulin: a hormone produced by the pancreas that is necessary for carbohydrate metabolism. It serves as the "key" to unlock the body's cells to allow carbohydrate to enter the cell to be burned for energy. Insulin influences the way we metabolize foods, determining whether we burn fat, protein, or carbohydrate to meet our energy needs, ultimately determining whether we will store fat.

Ketones: a waste product of abnormal fat metabolism, produced in the absence of carbohydrates as an energy source or by the insulin-deprived body; from fats being broken down to be used as an inefficient energy source. They accumulate in the blood, causing bad breath, frequent urination, interrupted sleep, constipation, nausea, general edginess, and lightheadedness.

Ketosis: a dangerous state of imbalance wherein the body is circulating high levels of acidic ketone waste products from fat being utilized as an inefficient energy source. Ketosis will be symptomized by all of the above symptoms of an accumulation of ketones. In the clearing of these ketones, the body excretes sodium and potassium, which can result in dehydration and abnormal heart rhythms. In dumping the ketones, the body retains uric acid, which can trigger gouty arthritis, gout, and kidney stones.

Lactase: enzyme that digests lactose

LH (luteinizing hormone): along with FSH, is produced in the pituitary gland to stimulate the rise of estrogen and progesterone during the menstrual cycle

Libido: sexual drive

Melatonin: light-sensitive, sleep-regulating hormone produced by the pineal gland.

Menstrual cycle: a woman's monthly reproductive cycle, with stimulation of the ovulation, corresponding hormone production and resultant thickening of the uterine lining, then the shedding of this lining as a menstrual period if pregnancy does not occur

Menopause: the point in time when menstruation stops permanently

Metabolism: how many calories we burn per minute for body functions—both automatic, involuntary functions like breathing, heart beat, digestion, and blood circulation, and through voluntary activity and movement. The largest amount of calories used (70 percent) are those burned to maintain our basic body functioning.

Migraines: headaches characterized by one-sided throbbing pain, nausea, and hypersensitivity to light and noise

Miso: soybean paste that is a combination of soybeans and a grain that is aged for one to three years

Muscle: a complex body system that uses energy to propel the body and body functions. Muscle stores glycogen and fatty acids to be used as energy.

Neuro-hormones: chemicals released in the brain that are natural painkillers and also help alleviate anxiety

Neurotransmitters: brain chemicals responsible for sending specialized messages from one brain cell to another. Examples are serotonin, endorphins, dopamine, and adenosine.

Norepinephrine: one of two primary stress response hormones, produced in the adrenal glands

Nutraceuticals: pharmacological agents in food that are vital for vibrant living

Osteoporosis: "brittle bone disease"; a reduction in bone mass and an increase in the porosity and fragility of the bone

Ovary: gland that produces eggs and all of the steroid hormones

Perimenopause: "around" the time of menopause when symptoms are occurring; may begin eight to ten years before the cessation of the menstrual cycle, but generally describes the period of time approximately two years before and two years after the final menstrual period

Phytoestrogens: plant hormones

Phytonutrients: chemicals in plants that give antioxidative and protective power to the body against disease. Examples are lycopene, carotene, and indoles.

PMS (premenstrual syndrome): physical and psychological/emotional symptoms associated with the post-ovulatory phase of the menstrual cycle. It is usually followed by a time entirely free of symptoms.

Premarin: conjugated equine estrogens, collected from a pregnant mare's urine

Prempro: drug containing combination of estrogen and progestin

Progesterone: hormone produced primarily in the ovaries that works with estrogen to prepare the uterine lining for implantation and growth of a baby

Progestin: synthetic version of progesterone

Prostaglandin: a group of naturally occurring fatty acids that stimulate contraction of the uterus and other smooth muscles. They have the ability to regulate acid secretion of the stomach, regulate temperature, control or cause inflammation, and also affect the action of certain hormones.

Protein: an essential nutrient that is part of the foods we eat — primarily animal products and legumes. It serves as a vital building block for the body for growth, healing, and repair and can be used as an energy source when carbohydrate intake is deficient.

SAD (seasonal affective disorder): a form of depression linked to inadequate exposure to light

Serotonin: a chemical neurotransmitter that brings calm, increased well-being, a bright perspective, a sense of satiety, and appetite control. Serotonin is called the master weight control drug because of its blocking of bingeing and increased appetite triggers.

Soy nuts: roasted mature soybeans

Steroid hormones: estrogen, progesterone, testosterone

Strength exercises: those exercises that tone, shape, and define muscles through repetitive movement against resistance

Stress incontinence: the loss of urine with coughing, sneezing, laughing, exercising, etc.

Tempeh: fermented mixture of whole soybeans and a grain

Testosterone: hormone that fuels sexual desire and enhances pleasure

Tofu: food made from curdled fresh soymilk

TriEst (triple natural estrogen): a chemical composition similar to what the body produces

Triglycerides: a body fat that serves to transport nutrients throughout the body. Triglycerides often rise to a high level in the blood when there is a nutrient overload (too much food at one time), a high intake of refined carbohydrates, or excessive intake of alcohol.

TSH (thyroid-stimulating hormone): hormone made by the pituitary gland that regulates the amount of thyroid hormone released into the blood

Tyrosine: amino acid that increases the production of dopamine and norepinephrine

Vaginitis: inflammation of vaginal tissues.

Vasomotor flushing: hot flash

WHI (Women's Health Initiative): U.S. government-sponsored program that published a study in 2002 showing significant increase in the risk of heart disease, breast cancer, and stroke among women on HRT

RECIPE INDEX

Subject Index

polyunsaturated, 206
saturated, 114, 206
fatty acids, essential. *See* essential fatty acids (EFA)
Femhrt, 64
fertility, 42
fiber, 57, 58, 109, 114, 166, 221–27, 234–35
fibrocystic disease, 238–39
fibroids, 19
fibromyalgia, 98
fight-or-flight response, 43, 221, 249
filtration, water, 201
fish, 92, 97, 108, 209
fish oil, 91, 97
fitness, 27, 72, 249, 252, 258
F.I.T.T., 259–60
flatulence, 113
flavonoids, 180
flavorings, 237
flaxseed, 69, 75, 97, 114, 187, 208, 209–11
flexibility, 258
fluid retention, 50, 56, 58, 199, 244
fluorescent light, 264
flushing, 37, 73
focus, 146
folic acid, 91, 223
follicle-stimulating hormone. *See* FSH
food. *See also* Recipes Index
    and hot flashes, 76
    high in B vitamins, 91
    high in fiber, 225
    high in phytoestrogen, 186
    high in protein, 167
    and memory, 90–93
    and overall health, 157
    processed, 237
    refined, 229

Food-Feelings-and-Findings Journal, 36–37, 137–40, 155, 183
food pyramid, 178
foreplay, 103
forgetfulness. *See* memory
Fosamax, 110
fractures, 62, 110
free radicals, 92, 180, 212
friendship, 154, 284–85, 286. *See also* relationships
fruits, 58, 109, 114, 177–84, 223, 234
FSH, 31, 33, 36, 74, 191
fuel gauge, 141
full-spectrum lights, 265
fuzzy thinking, *See* mental fuzziness

gallbladder disease, 114
gallstones, 114
gas, 35, 113, 115
gastrointestinal distress, 113
glucagon, 167, 168
glucose, 92, 159, 222, 230, 254
glycemic response, 222
goiter, 192
grains, refined, 221, 223–24
grains, whole, 57, 58, 76, 98, 109, 114, 126, 221–27
grapefruit, 93, 178, 180
green tea, 112, 239, 242

hair, 35, 58, 107–9
hair, facial, 45
HDL cholesterol, 191, 208, 211, 255
headaches, 35, 42, 45, 58, 78, 79, 117–19, 159, 196, 199, 207, 232, 240. *See also* migraines
heart attack, 63, 77, 196

irritability, 35, 50, 58, 96, 160, 238, 240

irritable bowel syndrome, 35, 113

isoflavones, 186, 187–88, 189, 190, 191, 192, 210

Japan, 97, 158, 186

java, 239, 240

jet lag, 86, 266

jogging, 112, 219, 252

joints, 35, 58

journal, 152, 155. *See also* Food-Feelings-and-Findings Journal

junk diet, 126

Kegel exercises, 104

kidneys, 112

K-Y, 103

lactase, 216, 217

lactose intolerance, 216–17

laughter, 99

laxative, 196

LDL cholesterol, 191, 208, 211

lean proteins, 159, 161, 164, 166, 190

lecithin, 92

legumes, 186, 223

lethargy, 34, 95, 240, 266

LH, 33

libido, 58, 101–6

licorice root, 78

light, 263–69. *See also* sunlight

light, natural, 84, 99

lignans, 187, 210

lipids, 191

love, 286

Loveless, Caron, 283–84

lovemaking, 99, 102, 105–6

lubricant, 102, 103

lunch, 166, 171–72. *See also* Recipes Index

lung disease, 180, 183

lutein, 109, 180

luteinizing hormone, 33

lycopene, 109, 180

macronutrients, 168

magnesium, 58, 77, 84, 91, 97–98, 111, 126, 170, 223

mangos, 77, 105

massage, 98

meals, 75, 84, 115, 126, 128, 159, 163, 164, 165, 240, 291, 294

meats, 93

medications, 85, 103

melatonin, 85, 86, 264

memory, 35, 58, 63, 64, 89–93, 250

men, 273–76

menopause, 25, 55–58, 60, 62. *See also* perimenopause

artificial, 26, 56

natural, 31

menstruation. *See* periods

mental attitude, 63

mental fuzziness, 24, 35, 58, 89–93, 195

metabolism, 58, 124–26, 164, 209, 249, 254

methylxanthines, 238–39

micronutrients, 168

migraines, 35, 97, 117–19. *See also* headaches

milk, 58, 111, 216

minerals, 169–70

mini-meals. *See* snacks

miso, 188, 189–90

monounsaturated fats, 206, 211–13

mood swings, 34, 35, 58, 95–99, 102, 244

We want to hear from you. Please send your comments about this book to us in care of zreview@zondervan.com. Thank you.

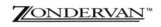

GRAND RAPIDS, MICHIGAN 49530 USA

WWW.ZONDERVAN.COM